# Physical Therapy Prescriptions for Musculoskeletal Disorders

# Physical Therapy Prescriptions for Musculoskeletal Disorders

**Grant C. Cooper, MD**
Princeton Spine and Joint Center, LLC
Princeton, New Jersey

**Evan Chait, PT**
Kinetic Physical Therapy
Ramsey, New Jersey

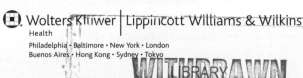

. Wolters Kluwer | Lippincott Williams & Wilkins
Health
Philadelphia · Baltimore · New York · London
Buenos Aires · Hong Kong · Sydney · Tokyo

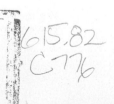

*Acquisitions Editor*: Robert Hurley
*Product Manager*: Elise M. Paxson
*Production Manager*: Bridgett Dougherty
*Senior Manufacturing Manager*: Benjamin Rivera
*Marketing Manager*: Lisa Lawrence
*Design Coordinator*: Doug Smock
*Production Service*: SPi Technologies

Printed in China

**Library of Congress Cataloging-in-Publication Data**
Cooper, Grant, M.D.
    Physical therapy prescriptions for musculoskeletal disorders / Grant C. Cooper, Evan Chait.
        p. ; cm.
    Includes bibliographical references and index.
    ISBN 978-1-60547-672-8 (alk. paper)
    1. Musculoskeletal system—Diseases—Physical therapy—Case studies.  I. Chait, Evan.  II. Title.
    [DNLM: 1. Musculoskeletal Diseases—diagnosis—Case Reports. 2. Musculoskeletal Diseases—therapy—Case Reports. 3. Musculoskeletal System—injuries—Case Reports. 4. Pain—therapy—Case Reports. 5. Physical Therapy Modalities—Case Reports. WE 140]

    RC925.5C664 2010
    616.7'062—dc22

                                                                                        2010030538

DISCLAIMER
Care has been taken to confirm the accuracy of the information presented and to describe generally accepted practices. However, the authors, editors, and publisher are not responsible for errors or omissions or for any consequences from application of the information in this book and make no warranty, expressed or implied, with respect to the currency, completeness, or accuracy of the contents of the publication. Application of the information in a particular situation remains the professional responsibility of the practitioner.

The authors, editors, and publisher have exerted every effort to ensure that drug selection and dosage set forth in this text are in accordance with current recommendations and practice at the time of publication. However, in view of ongoing research, changes in government regulations, and the constant flow of information relating to drug therapy and drug reactions, the reader is urged to check the package insert for each drug for any change in indications and dosage and for added warnings and precautions. This is particularly important when the recommended agent is a new or infrequently employed drug.

Some drugs and medical devices presented in the publication have Food and Drug Administration (FDA) clearance for limited use in restricted research settings. It is the responsibility of the health care provider to ascertain the FDA status of each drug or device planned for use in their clinical practice.

To purchase additional copies of this book, call our customer service department at (800) 638—3030 or fax orders to (301) 223—2320. International customers should call (301) 223—2300.

Visit Lippincott Williams & Wilkins on the Internet: at LWW.com. Lippincott Williams & Wilkins customer service representatives are available from 8:30 am to 6 pm, EST.

10 9 8 7 6 5 4 3 2 1

CCS1110

*For Ana and Mila*

# ACKNOWLEDGMENTS

First and foremost, I would like to thank my wife Jen who is my inspiration and strength, and without her patience, this book would have not been possible. My thanks to my daughter Joline, who lights up my day by her funny antics and brings joy to our household.

Thank you to Eric Van Pelt who vigorously worked on the pictures for the book; his commitment to the creation of the book was exceptional. Special thanks to all the physicians I have learned from, for entrusting your patients in my hands over the years. Without this trust, the ideas in this book would only be theoretical and not practically based.

Thank you to my best friend Karen Shirazi and her husband Brian McGowan, whose loyalty and faith are unshakeable. Thank you for taking care of business in the good and bad times.

Thank you to my parents for all your love and support over the years. Lastly, thank you to my team at Kinetic Physical Therapy; you are an extraordinary and a gifted group of talented people.

—Evan Chait

# CONTENTS

# PART **1**

## CERVICAL DISORDERS

# CASE 1

## MYOFASCIAL NECK PAIN

**CC:** Neck pain

**HPI:** Ms. P is 36 years old and presents with 4 months of axial neck and bilateral trapezius pain. She says the pain does not travel into her shoulders or arms, and she denies any numbness, tingling, burning, or weakness. The pain is present all the time and worse toward the end of the day. On a scale of 0 to 10 (with 0 being no pain and 10 being unbearable pain), she says the pain is 4 at present and can get as bad as 7 or 8 at the end of the day. Ms. P works as an administrator and spends lots of time in front of her computer and on the phone. She has not had a formal ergonomic evaluation at work but says she does use a headset.

This is the first time that Ms. P is coming to the doctor for this problem. She has not had any imaging studies and has not been to physical therapy. She occasionally takes Advil for the pain and finds this mildly helpful.

**PMHx:** None

**PSHx:** None

**Meds:** Advil prn; oral contraceptives

**Allergies:** NKDA

**Social:** No tobacco; social EtOH

**ROS:** Noncontributory

## PHYSICAL EXAM

Ms. P is a well-developed, well-nourished female NAD who looks her stated age. BP: 116/68, P: 72, RR: 14. She has 5/5 strength, intact sensation, and 2+ biceps, triceps, and brachioradialis reflexes in her upper extremities bilaterally. She has full range of motion of her neck, with pain at the end range of motion in all directions except flexion. Her cervical paraspinals, trapezius, and rhomboids are tight and tender bilaterally. No specific trigger points are identifiable. 2+ distal pulses are palpated bilaterally.

### Impression

Myofascial neck pain

### Plan

1. X-rays to rule out any underlying structural abnormality
2. Physical therapy

## PHYSICAL THERAPY

The patient is a 36-year-old female referred to physical therapy for the treatment of myofascial neck pain that started 4 months ago with an insidious onset. No radicular symptoms are noted.

**PMHx:** as above
**Diagnostics:** as above
**Meds:** as above
**Occupation:** administrator
**Pain scale:** 4–7–8/10 pain
**Increase pain:** prolonged sitting >20 minutes; C/S rotation; C/S extension; stress; carrying anything >10 lb; cold drafts
**Decrease pain:** hot showers; walking

### Range of Motion

**Cervical spine**
R rotation: WNL pain at end range
L rotation: WNL pain at end range
Extension: WNL pain at end range
Flexion: WNL
R sidebending: 50% limited with tightness
L sidebending: 50% limited with tightness

*Assisted shoulder shrug decreased pain and tightness and normalized sidebending

**Thoracic spine**
Hyperkyphotic position note
Decreased T/S reversal with wall arm raise
Decreased T/S rotation with pectoralis major restriction

**Joint play**
Thoracic spine: T7/6/5 2/6 with firm end feel
**Special tests**
Spurling test +
Compression test +
**Manual muscle testing**
Bilateral mid trapezius—4–/5
**Tight tender points/soft tissue restrictions**
Bilateral upper trapezius—trigger points
Bilateral levator scapulae—trigger points
Bilateral serrratus posterior superior and spinalis thoracis/longissimus thoracis—myofascial adhesions
Bilateral pectoralis major—myofascial restriction
**Ergonomics**
Poor ergonomics noted

## ASSESSMENT

The patient presents with significant myofascial restrictions located in the serratus posterior superior and pectoralis major and trigger points in upper trapezius and levator scapulae. Poor ergonomics and poor-fair thoracic mobility are contributing to the patient's pain patterns. Pectoralis major restrictions combined with decreased T/S rotation are limiting T/S reversal.

### Plan

Self–myofascial release/corrective flexibility/corrective exercises/corrective manual therapy/modalities

### Self–Myofascial Release

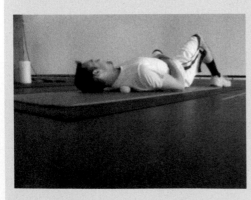

**FIGURE 1.1A**. Tennis ball roll: bilateral upper/mid trapezius.

(*continued*)

## Self–Myofascial Release (*continued*)

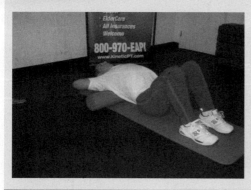

**FIGURE 1.1B.** Foam roll: perpendicular from T5-7.

## Corrective Flexibility

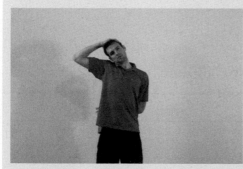

**FIGURE 1.2A.** Static: bilateral upper trapezius.

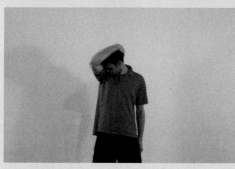

**FIGURE 1.2B.** Static: bilateral levator scapulae.

(*continued*)

## Corrective Flexibility (*continued*)

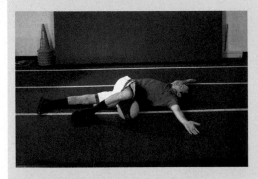

**FIGURE 1.2C.** Static: sideline T/S rotation with pectoralis major bilateral.

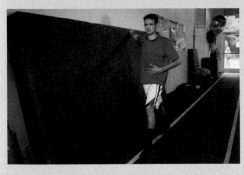

**FIGURE 1.2D.** Active: standing pectoralis major with T/S rotation/split stance position.

## Corrective Exercise

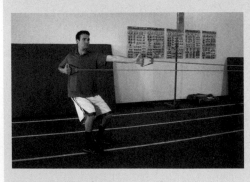

**FIGURE 1.3A.** Pull: parallel stance/ theraband/total body rotation.

(*continued*)

## Corrective Exercise (*continued*)

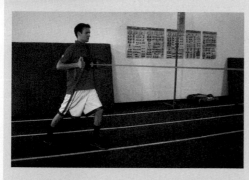

**FIGURE 1.3B.** Pull: split stance/ theraband/two arms.

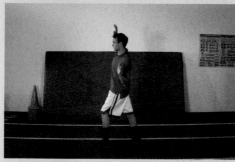

**FIGURE 1.3C.** Walk matrix.

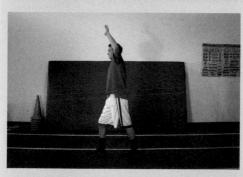

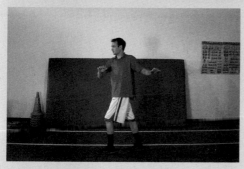

(*continued*)

## Corrective Exercise (*continued*)

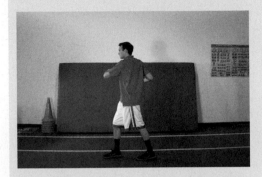

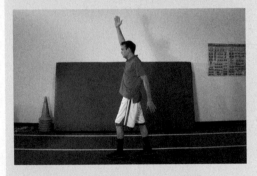

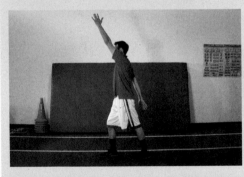

## Manual Therapy

1. Warming technique: bilateral upper/mid trapezius; levator scapulae; posterior elements from C1-T1
2. Inhibitory technique: bilateral upper trapezius/suboccipitals
3. Elongation technique: bilateral levator scapulae; serratus posterior superior and T/S erectors
4. Static stretch: T/S rotation with pectoralis major in sideline
5. PA mobilizations to T5-7

## Modalities: prn

1. Moist heat
2. Continuous US

Orthopedic and Rehabilitation Associates
Orthopedic Street
Omaha, OH
(555) 555-5555
Fax. (666) 666-7777

PATIENT: _Ms. P_
DATE: _2009_

## ORTHOPAEDIC REHABILITATION PRESCRIPTION

| *REHAB THERAPIES* | ☒ PT | ☐ OT | ☐ SESSIONS/WK _2_ |
|---|---|---|---|

TOTAL _12_

☒ NEW DIAGNOSIS    ☐ RE-EVALUATION    ☒ OUTPATIENT

DIAGNOSIS1 _Myofascial Neck Pain_
　ICD _____

DIAGNOSIS2 _____
　ICD _____

PREGNANT? ☐ YES ☒ NO    PERTINENTMEDICALHISTORY: _None_

GOALS:
MD/DO: ☒ INCREASE MOBILITY ☒ INCREASE ADL ☒ INCREASE STRENGTH ☒ DECREASE PAIN

PRECAUTIONS: ☐ CARDIAC    MAX-SBP _____ DBP _____ HR _____
ABOVE BASELINE    ☐ DIABETES: HYPER/HYPOGLYCEMIA ☐ ORTHOSTASIS
☐ OTHER _____
WEIGHT BEARING:    ☐ WBAT    ☐ TTWB    ☐ NWB
　TO: _____
MODALITIES: ☐ ULTRASOUND TO: _1.2 W/CM2 x 7 Min to cervical paraspinals B/L_
　　　　　☐ E-STIM    TO: _X 7 min to cervical paraspinals_
B/L _____
　☐ FLUID THERAPY    ☐ JOBST    ☐ PARAFFIN
　TO: _____
　☐ ICE    TO: _10 min to cervical paraspinals_
B/L _____
　☐ HOTPACKS    TO: _10 min to cervical paraspinals B/L_
　☐ EXERCISES ☐ PROM ☐ AAROM ☐ AROM
　TO: _____
　☒ PRE's ☐ ISOMETRICS ☐ ISOKINETICS
　TO: _____
　☐ SLIDEBOARD ☐ PLYOMETRICS ☐ MODIFIED KNEE BEND
☐ STEPUPS
☐ LUMBAR STABILIZATION ☐ WILLIAM's ☐ McKENZIE ☒ CERVICAL EXERCISES
☐ RELAXATION ☐ COORDINATIONa
MANUAL: ☒ CONTRACT RELAX ☐ CRANIOSACRAL ☒ JONES/C-STRAIN ☒ SOFT
TISSUE MOBILIZATION
　☒ STRETCHING ☒ MASSAGE ☒ MYOF AS RELEASE ☒ SPRAY/STRETCH
　TO: _Cervical paraspinals_
EDUCATION: ☒ MOBILITY: ☐ TRANSFERS ☒ ADL ☒ HEP ☒ ENERGY CONSERV
　☐ WORK HARDENING ☒ BIOMECHANICS ☐ 1
HANDED TECHNIQUES
　☐ GAIT TRAINING ☐ FINE MOTOR ☐ COORD/BALANCE
OTHER: _____
_____

The above is medically necessary to decrease debility and achieve ADL independence. Also to:
☐ decrease pain, ☐ improve strength/endurance, ☐ improve balance coordination, ☐ improve gait,
☐ improve transfers,
Other _____

PHYSICIAN'S SIGNATURE _____    DATE _____

# CASE **2**

## CERVICAL RADICULITIS

**CC:** Neck and right arm pain

**HPI:** Mr. X is a 53-year-old investment banker who complains of 4 weeks of neck pain. In the last 2 weeks, the pain has started radiating down his arm. The pain radiates down the posterior upper arm and travels into the hand. He denies any numbness, tingling, or burning. He has been taking 400 mg of Ibuprofen every 6 hours for 3 days and says he feels "a little better." The pain is rated as 4/10 intensity on average. It is worse when he uses the phone. He has not had any imaging studies and has not gone to physical therapy.

**PMHx:** HTN

**PSHx:** Appendectomy; R knee meniscectomy

**Meds:** Advil prn; HCTZ

**Allergies:** Sulfa gives him a rash

**Social:** No tobacco; social EtOH

**ROS:** Noncontributory

## PHYSICAL EXAMINATION

On exam, Mr. X is a well-developed man who looks younger than his stated age. BP: 128/78, P: 80, RR: 14. He has 5/5 strength, intact sensation, and 2+ biceps, triceps, and brachioradialis reflexes in his upper extremities bilaterally. His cervical paraspinals, trapezius, and rhomboids are tight and tender bilaterally; right greater than left. No specific trigger points are identifiable. He has full range of motion of his neck,

**11**

with pain at the end range of bilateral rotation and lateral flexion. He has a positive Spurling's on the right that reproduces his arm symptoms. 2+ distal pulses are palpated bilaterally.

## Impression

Right cervical radiculitis

## Plan

1. X-rays to rule out any underlying structural abnormality.
2. Instruction to start using a headset instead of cradling his phone inbetween his ear and shoulder.
3. Physical therapy.
4. Meloxicam 15 mg PO daily #14

# PHYSICAL THERAPY

The patient is a 53-year-old male who complains of neck pain that started 4 weeks ago. In the last 2 weeks, the pain has started radiating down the posterior aspect of the arm into the hand.

**PMHx:** as above

**Diagnostics:** as above

**Meds:** as above

**Occupation:** investment banker

**Pain scale:** 4/10 pain

**Increase pain:** talking on the phone; prolonged sitting >30 minutes; C/S rotation right great than left; C/S extension; stress; carrying anything >10 lb; cold drafts

**Decrease pain:** hot showers; rotating his head left with C/S flexion

## Range of Motion

**Cervical spine**
R rotation: WNL pain with symptoms into the right hand
L rotation: WNL
Extension: WNL pain with symptoms into the right hand
Flexion: WNL
R sidebending: 50% limited with pain and symptoms into the right hand
L sidebending: WNL
**Thoracic spine**
Hyperkyphotic position note
Normal T/S reversal with wall arm raise noted
**Joint play**
Thoracic spine: WNL
C/S spine: WNL

**Special tests**
Spurling's +
C/S distraction decreased symptoms
Scalene compression –
**Manual muscle testing**
WNL
**Neurodynamic assessment**
Radial nerve glide diminished
**Tight tender points/soft tissue restrictions**
Bilateral upper trapezius—trigger points
Right levator scapulae—trigger points
Right serratus posterior superior and spinalis thoracis/longissimus thoracis—myofascial adhesions
Right longus capitis—myofascial adhesions
**Ergonomics**
Poor ergonomics noted

## ASSESSMENT

The patient presents with right side facet joint inflammation that compresses the posterior cord of the brachial plexus with right cervical rotation, right sidebending, and during the Spurling test. C/S traction decreases the symptoms. Myofascial restrictions located in the right serratus posterior superior and right longus capitis and trigger points in bilateral upper trapezius and right levator scapulae. Poor ergonomics and diminished neurodynamic capabilities noted.

### Plan

Self–myofascial release/corrective flexibility/corrective exercises/corrective manual therapy/modalities

### Self–Myofascial Release

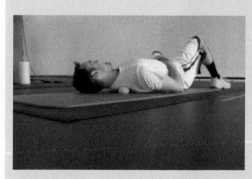

**FIGURE 2.1A.** Tennis ball roll: bilateral upper/levator scapulae.

## Corrective Flexibility

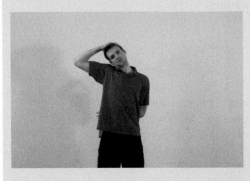

**FIGURE 2.2A.** Static: right upper trapezius.

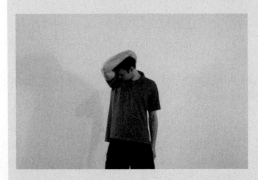

**FIGURE 2.2B.** Static: right levator scapulae.

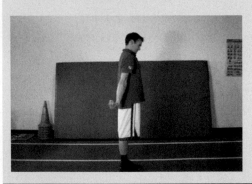

**FIGURE 2.2C.** Neurodynamic: right radial nerve.

## Corrective Exercise

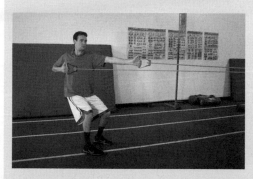

**FIGURE 2.3A.** Pull: parallel stance/ theraband/total body rotation.

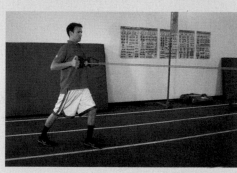

**FIGURE 2.3B.** Pull: split stance/ theraband/two arms.

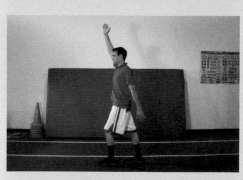

**FIGURE 2.3C.** Walk matrix.

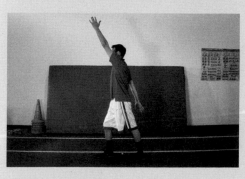

(*continued*)

## Corrective Exercise (*continued*)

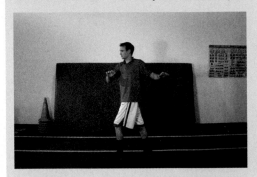

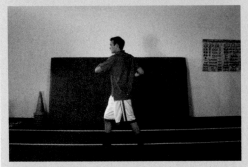

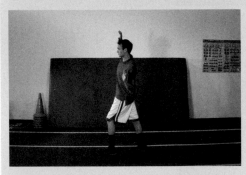

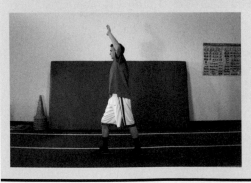

## Manual Therapy

1. Warming technique: bilateral upper/mid trapezius; levator scapulae; posterior elements from C1-T1
2. Inhibitory technique: bilateral upper trapezius/suboccipitals
3. Elongation technique: right levator scapulae; serratus posterior superior and T/S erectors; longus capitis
4. Neuromobilization: right radial nerve
5. C/S traction (manual or mechanical)

## Modalities: prn

1. Moist heat
2. US pulsed

Orthopedic and Rehabilitation Associates
Orthopedic Street
Omaha, OH
(555) 555-5555
Fax. (666) 666-7777

PATIENT: _Mr. X_
DATE: _2009_

## ORTHOPAEDIC REHABILITATION PRESCRIPTION

*REHAB THERAPIES* ☒ PT ☐ OT ☐ SESSIONS/WK _2_
TOTAL _12_

☒ NEW DIAGNOSIS ☐ RE-EVALUATION ☒ OUTPATIENT

DIAGNOSIS1 _Cervical radiculitis_
   ICD _____

DIAGNOSIS2 _____
   ICD _____

PREGNANT? ☐ YES ☐ NO      PERTINENTMEDICALHISTORY: _None_

GOALS:
MD/DO: ☒ INCREASE MOBILITY ☒ INCREASE ADL ☒ INCREASE STRENGTH ☒ DECREASE PAIN

PRECAUTIONS: ☒ CARDIAC    MAX-SBP _20_ DBP _10_ HR _20_
ABOVE BASELINE    ☐ DIABETES: HYPER/HYPOGLYCEMIA ☐ ORTHOSTASIS
☐ OTHER _____

WEIGHT BEARING: ☐ WBAT ☐ TTWB ☐ NWB
   TO: _____
MODALITIES: ☐ ULTRASOUND TO: _1.2 W/CM2 x 1 Min to cervical paraspinals B/L_
      ☐ E-STIM    TO: _X 1 min to cervical paraspinals_
B/L _____
      ☐ FLUID THERAPY    ☐ JOBST    ☐ PARAFFIN
   TO: _____
      ☐ ICE    TO: _10 min to cervical paraspinals_
B/L _____
      ☐ HOTPACKS    TO: _10 min to cervical paraspinals B/L_
      ☐ EXERCISES ☐ PROM ☐ AAROM ☐ AROM
   TO: _____
      ☒ PRE's ☐ ISOMETRICS ☐ ISOKINETICS
   TO: _____
      ☐ SLIDEBOARD ☐ PLYOMETRICS ☐ MODIFIED KNEE BEND
☐ STEPUPS
☐ LUMBAR STABILIZATION ☐ WILLIAM's ☐ McKENZIE ☒ CERVICAL EXERCISES
☐ RELAXATION ☐ COORDINATION
MANUAL: ☒ CONTRACT RELAX ☐ CRANIOSACRAL ☒ JONES/C-STRAIN ☒ SOFT
TISSUE MOBILIZATION
      ☒ STRETCHING ☒ MASSAGE ☒ MYOF AS RELEASE ☒ SPRAY/STRETCH
   TO: _Cervicalparaspinals_
EDUCATION: ☒ MOBILITY: ☐ TRANSFERS ☒ ADL ☒ HEP ☐ ENERGY CONSERV
☐ WORK HARDENING ☒ BIOMECHANICS ☐ 1
HANDED TECHNIQUES
☐ GAIT TRAINING ☐ FINE MOTOR ☐ COORD/BALANCE
OTHER: _____
_____

The above is medically necessary to decrease debility and achieve ADL independence. Also to:
☒ decrease pain, ☒ improve strength/endurance, ☒ improve balance coordination, ☐ improve gait,
☐ improve transfers,
Other _____

PHYSICIAN'S SIGNATURE _____ DATE _____

# CASE **3**

# WHIPLASH INJURY

**CC:** Neck pain

**HPI:** Ms. L is 44 years old and has had neck pain for the last 3 months ever since being involved in a motor vehicle accident in which she was a driver of a car that was rear-ended at a stop light. She had gone to the emergency room and the x-rays of her neck and thoracic spine at that time were normal, per the patient. She does not have her x-rays with her and says it would be difficult to get them because the accident occurred out of state and she does not want to go back there. Ms. L felt okay the day after the injury but subsequently developed axial neck pain that occasionally travels into the top of her head. She denies any radiating symptoms to her upper extremities. She denies any numbness, tingling, burning, or weakness. The pain sometimes keeps her awake at night when her neck goes into spasms. She rates the pain as 3/10 at its best and 7/10 at its worst.

**PMHx:** None

**PSHx:** Laparoscopic cholecystectomy

**Meds:** Advil prn

**Allergies:** NKDA

**Social:** No tobacco; no EtOH

**ROS:** Noncontributory

# PHYSICAL EXAMINATION

On exam, Ms. L is an overweight woman who appears her stated age. BP: 118/60, P: 70, RR: 15. She has 5/5 strength, intact sensation, and 2+ biceps, triceps, and brachioradialis reflexes in her upper extremities bilaterally. Her cervical paraspinals, trapezius, and rhomboids are tight and tender bilaterally; left greater than right. No specific trigger points are identifiable. She has full range of motion of her neck. She has pain when extending her neck and with oblique extension to the left. Spurling's is negative. 2+ distal pulses are palpated bilaterally.

## Impression

Whiplash syndrome with likely z-joint pain.

## Plan

1. X-rays to evaluate the facets.
2. Physical therapy.
3. Flexeril 5 mg PO bedtime prn #30

# PHYSICAL THERAPY

The patient is a 44-year-old female who presents with axial neck pain that started 3 months ago following an MVA. She was hit from behind. The patient has had no physical therapy treatment previously and was referred to physical therapy to treat whiplash. Pain is constant.

**PMHx:** as above

**Diagnostics:** as above

**Meds:** as above

**Occupation:** housewife

**Pain scale:** 3/10 pain at rest up to 7/10

**Increase pain:** pain is constant; C/S rotation; driving; carrying daughter

**Decrease pain:** ice; muscle relaxers

## Range of Motion

**Cervical spine**
R rotation: WNL with apprehension and pain
L rotation: WNL with apprehension and pain
Extension: WNL with apprehension and pain
Flexion: WNL with apprehension and pain
R sidebending: 75% limited with apprehension and pain
L sidebending: 75% limited with apprehension and pain
**Thoracic spine**
WNL

**Joint play**
C2/3 2/6 bilateral
C3/4-2/6 bilateral
**Special tests**
Spurling's –
Vertebral artery test –
Alar ligament test –
**Manual muscle testing**
WNL
**Neurodynamic assessment**
Great occipital nerve entrapment noted at the superior nuchal line of the upper trapezius attachment. Referral to forehead.
**Tight tender points/soft tissue restrictions**
Bilateral upper trapezius—trigger points
Bilateral levator scapulae—trigger points
Bilateral longus coli—trigger points
Bilateral rectus capitis major/minor and superior/inferior obliquus capitis—trigger points
Bilateral longus capitis—myofascial adhesions
Bilateral scalenes—myofascial adhesions
**Ergonomics**
WNL

## ASSESSMENT

The patient presents with significant soft tissue restrictions in the bilateral longus coli, suboccipitals, and scalenes. Joint restrictions are noted at the upper cervicals from C2-4 secondary to soft tissue restrictions. Trigger points found in the upper trapezius and suboccipitals referred a headache to the forehead along with greater occipital nerve entrapment where the upper trapezius attaches to the superior nuchal line.

### Plan

Self–myofascial release/corrective flexibility/corrective exercises/corrective manual therapy/modalities

## Self Myofascial Release

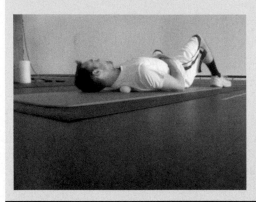

**FIGURE 3.1.** Tennis ball roll: bilateral upper/levator scapulae.

## Corrective Flexibility

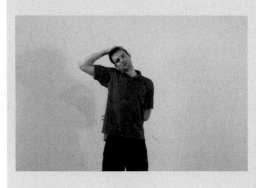

**FIGURE 3.2A.** Static: bilateral upper trapezius.

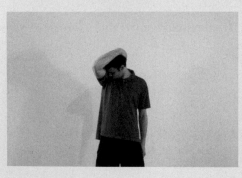

**FIGURE 3.2B.** Static: bilateral levator scapulae.

(*continued*)

## Corrective Flexibility (*continued*)

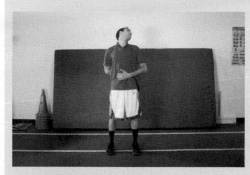

**FIGURE 3.2C.** Static: bilateral scalenes.

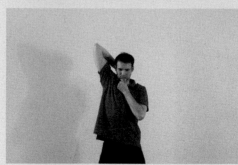

**FIGURE 3.2D.** Static: bilateral suboccipitals.

## Corrective Exercise

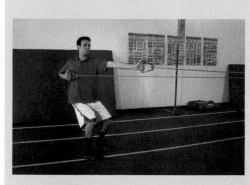

**FIGURE 3.3A.** Pull: parallel stance/theraband/total body rotation.

(*continued*)

## Corrective Exercise (*continued*)

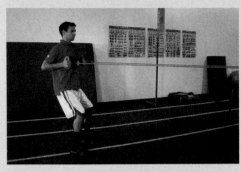

**FIGURE 3.3B.** Pull: split stance/theraband/two arms.

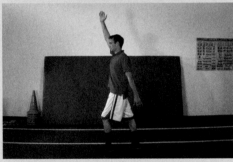

**FIGURE 3.3C.** Walk matrix.

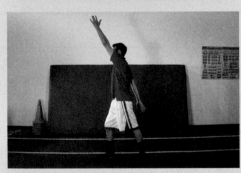

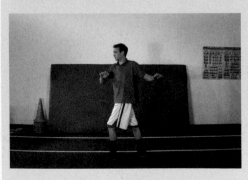

(*continued*)

## Corrective Exercise (*continued*)

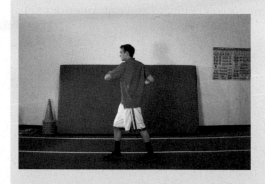

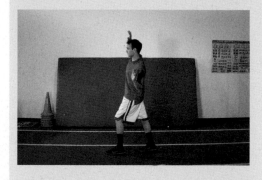

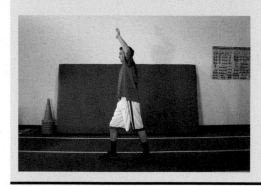

## Manual Therapy

1. Warming technique: bilateral upper/mid trapezius; levator scapulae, posterior elements from C1-T1
2. Inhibitory technique. bilateral upper trapezius/suboccipitals/ longus coli

3. Elongation technique: bilateral upper trapezius; longus coli; longus capitis
4. Neuromobilization: bilateral greater occipital nerve at superior nuchal line

## Modalities: prn

1. Ice pack
2. US pulsed

Orthopedic and Rehabilitation Associates
Orthopedic Street
Omaha, OH
(555) 555-5555
Fax. (666) 666-7777

PATIENT: _Ms. L_
DATE: _2009_

## ORTHOPAEDIC REHABILITATION PRESCRIPTION

**REHAB THERAPIES**  ☒ PT   ☐ OT   ☐ SESSIONS/WK _2_
TOTAL _12_

☒ NEW DIAGNOSIS   ☐ RE-EVALUATION   ☒ OUTPATIENT

DIAGNOSIS1 _Whiplash syndrome_
ICD _____

DIAGNOSIS2 _Neck pain_
ICD _____

PREGNANT? ☐ YES  ☒ NO   PERTINENTMEDICALHISTORY: _None_

GOALS:
MD/DO: ☒ INCREASE MOBILITY  ☒ INCREASE ADL  ☒ INCREASE STRENGTH  ☒ DECREASE PAIN

PRECAUTIONS: ☐ CARDIAC   MAX-SBP____ DBP____ HR____
ABOVE BASELINE   ☐ DIABETES: HYPER/HYPOGLYCEMIA  ☐ ORTHOSTASIS
☐ OTHER _____

WEIGHT BEARING:  ☐ WBAT   ☐ TTWB   ☐ NWB
TO: _____

MODALITIES: ☐ ULTRASOUND TO: _1.2 W/CM2 x 1 Min to cervical paraspinals B/L_
    ☐ E-STIM    TO: _x 1 min to cervical paraspinals_
B/L _____
    ☐ FLUID THERAPY   ☐ JOBST   ☐ PARAFFIN
    TO: _____
    ☐ ICE   TO: _10 min to cervical paraspinals_
B/L _____
    ☐ HOTPACKS   TO: _10 min to cervical paraspinals B/L_
    ☐ EXERCISES  ☐ PROM  ☐ AAROM  ☐ AROM
    TO: _____
    ☒ PRE's  ☐ ISOMETRICS  ☐ ISOKINETICS
    TO: _____
    ☐ SLIDEBOARD  ☐ PLYOMETRICS  ☐ MODIFIED KNEE BEND
☐ STEPUPS
☐ LUMBAR STABILIZATION  ☐ WILLIAM's  ☐ McKENZIE  ☒ CERVICAL EXERCISES
☐ RELAXATION  ☐ COORDINATION
MANUAL: ☒ CONTRACT RELAX  ☐ CRANIOSACRAL  ☒ JONES/C-STRAIN  ☒ SOFT
TISSUE MOBILIZATION
    ☒ STRETCHING ☒ MASSAGE ☒ MYOF AS RELEASE ☐ SPRAY/STRETCH
    TO: _Cervical paraspinals_
EDUCATION: ☒ MOBILITY: ☐ TRANSFERS ☒ ADL  ☒ HEP ☐ ENERGY CONSERV
☐ WORK HARDENING ☒ BIOMECHANICS ☐ 1
HANDED TECHNIQUES
☐ GAIT TRAINING ☐ FINE MOTOR ☐ COORD/BALANCE
OTHER: _____
_____

The above is medically necessary to decrease debility and achieve ADL independence. Also to:
☒ decrease pain, ☒ improve strength/endurance, ☒ improve balance coordination, ☐ improve gait,
☐ improve transfers,
Other _____

PHYSICIAN'S SIGNATURE _____   DATE _____

# CASE 4

# CHRONIC NECK PAIN

**CC:** Neck pain

**HPI:** Ms. J is 82 years old and has had neck pain for over 20 years. The pain does not radiate down her arms. She denies any numbness, tingling, burning, or weakness. She denies any trauma. Several years ago, she went to physical therapy for a few weeks and felt a little better but never learned her home exercise program and does not exercise at home. She presents today because, she says, the pain has gotten somewhat worse and she figured it was time to do something about it. She has not had any imaging studies in the last several years. She takes Tylenol prn for pain, which helps a little. The pain is rated as 4/10 intensity.

**PMHx:** HTN, high cholesterol, DM type II

**PSHx:** Cataract surgery

**Meds:** Toprol, Crestor, Glucophage, Tylenol prn

**Allergies:** NKDA

**Social:** No tobacco; social EtOH

**ROS:** Noncontributory

## PHYSICAL EXAMINATION

On exam, Ms. J is a well-developed woman who looks her stated age. BP: 144/88, P: 73, RR: 14. She has a kyphotic posture and 5/5 strength, intact sensation, and 2+ biceps, triceps, and brachioradialis reflexes in her upper extremities bilaterally. Her cervical paraspinals are tender bilaterally. A trigger point is elicited in the right trapezius that refers pain to the head. She has a negative Spurling's bilaterally. Her neck pain is worse with extension. She has slightly decreased range of motion of the neck in lateral flexion and rotation. 2+ distal pulses are palpated bilaterally.

## Impression

Chronic neck pain, likely secondary to z-joint arthritis

**Plan**

1. X-rays to evaluate the facet joints
2. Physical therapy

# PHYSICAL THERAPY

The patient is an 82-year-old female who presents with chronic neck pain that started over 20 years ago. Pain is from an insidious onset. Recently, the patient saw her medical doctor who referred her to physical therapy with a diagnosis of osteoarthritis in the cervical spine.

**Scale:** 4/10 pain

**Increase pain:** C/S extension; C/S rotation; C/S sidebending; prolonged sitting; cold weather

**Decrease pain:** warm weather; after showering; walking

## Range of Motion

**Cervical spine**
R rotation: 50% limited
L rotation: 50% limited
Extension: 75% limited with pain
Flexion: WNL with upper trapezius tightness
R sidebending: 75% limited
L sidebending: 75% limited

**Thoracic spine**
R rotation 50% limited no pectoralis
L rotation 50% limited no pectoralis
Hyperkyphosis

**Joint play**
2/6 bilateral all C/S segments
2/6 T3-6

**Special tests**
Spurling's –
Compression test –
Wall shoulder flexion test + (decreased T/S reversal)

**Manual muscle testing**
Middle trapezius bilateral 4/5
Rhomboids bilateral 3/5

**Neurodynamic assessment**
None

**Tight tender points/soft tissue restrictions**
Bilateral upper trapezius—trigger points
Bilateral mid trapezius—trigger points
Bilateral longus coli—trigger points
Bilateral spinalis thoracis; iliocostalis thoracis; longissumus thoracis
Bilateral scalenes—myofascial adhesions
**Ergonomics**
Poor

## ASSESSMENT

The patient presents with significant soft tissue restrictions in the bilateral longus coli, mid trapezius, upper trapezius, thoracic erectors, and scalenes. Joint restrictions are noted in C1-7 and poor T/S reversal and T/S rotation. Muscle weakness noted in bilateral middle trapezius and rhomboids of 4/5.

### Plan

Self–myofascial release/corrective flexibility/corrective exercises/corrective manual therapy/modalities

### Self–Myofascial Release

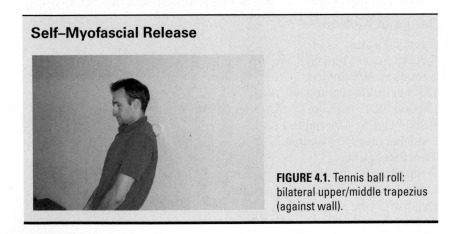

**FIGURE 4.1.** Tennis ball roll: bilateral upper/middle trapezius (against wall).

## Corrective Flexibility

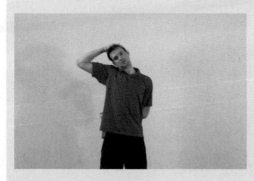

FIGURE 4.2A. Static: bilateral upper trapezius.

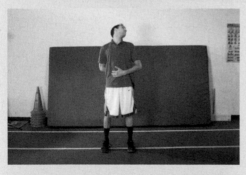

FIGURE 4.2B. Static: bilateral levator scapulae.

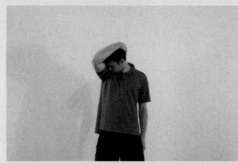

FIGURE 4.2C. Static: bilateral scalenes.

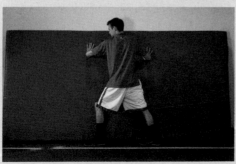

FIGURE 4.2D. Active: T/S rotation (against wall) no pectoralis major.

## Corrective Exercise

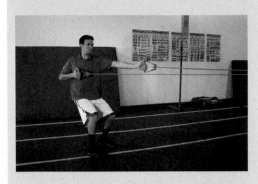

**FIGURE 4.3A.** Pull: parallel stance/theraband/total body rotation.

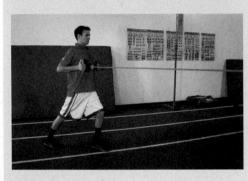

**FIGURE 4.3B.** Pull: split stance/ theraband/two arms.

(*continued*)

## Corrective Exercise (*continued*)

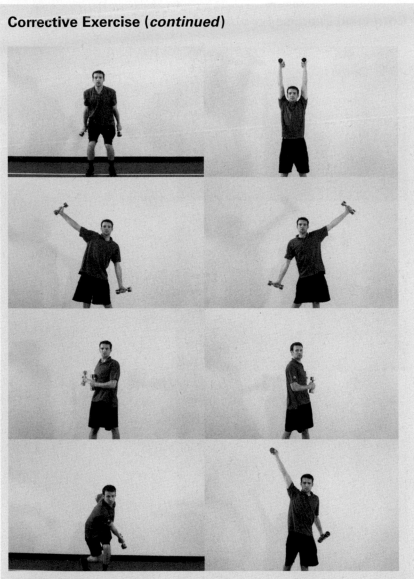

**FIGURE 4.3C.** Shoulder matrix.

(*continued*)

## Corrective Exercise (*continued*)

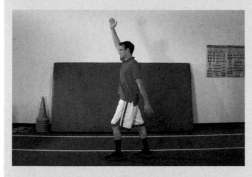

**FIGURE 4.3D.** Walk matrix.

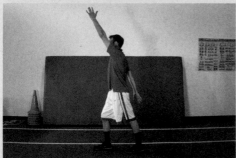

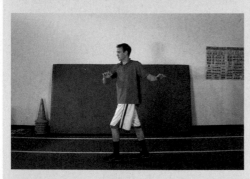

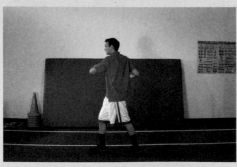

(*continued*)

## Corrective Exercise (*continued*)

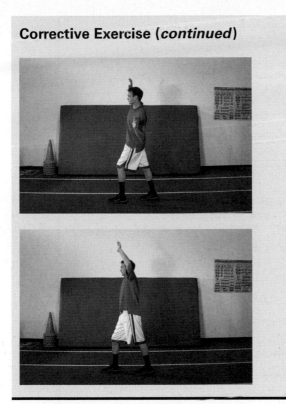

## Manual Therapy

1. Warming technique: bilateral upper/mid trapezius; levator scapulae; posterior elements from C1-T1
2. Inhibitory technique: bilateral upper trapezius/suboccipitals/middle trapezius
3. Elongation technique: bilateral upper trapezius
4. Joint mobilization techniques: T3-6 (Grade 1–3 PA mobilization)

## Modalities: prn

1. Hot pack
2. US continuous

## Home Exercise Program

1. Flexibility as above
2. Moist heat

Orthopedic and Rehabilitation Associates
Orthopedic Street
Omaha, OH
(555) 555-5555
Fax. (666) 666-7777

PATIENT: _Ms. J_
DATE: _2009_

### ORTHOPAEDIC REHABILITATION PRESCRIPTION

| *REHAB THERAPIES* | ☒ PT | ☐ OT | ☐ SESSIONS/WK _2_ |
| --- | --- | --- | --- |

TOTAL _12_

☒ NEW DIAGNOSIS    ☐ RE-EVALUATION    ☒ OUTPATIENT

DIAGNOSIS1 _Z-joint arthritis_
   ICD _____

DIAGNOSIS2 _Neck Pain_
   ICD _____

PREGNANT? ☐ YES ☒ NO     PERTINENTMEDICALHISTORY: _HTN, DM_

GOALS:
MD/DO: ☒ INCREASE MOBILITY ☒ INCREASE ADL ☒ INCREASE STRENGTH ☒ DECREASE PAIN

PRECAUTIONS: ☒ CARDIAC    MAX-SBP _20_ DBP _10_ HR _20_
ABOVE BASELINE   ☒ DIABETES: HYPER/HYPOGLYCEMIA ☐ ORTHOSTASIS
☐ OTHER _____

WEIGHT BEARING: ☐ WBAT ☐ TTWB ☐ NWB
   TO: _____

MODALITIES: ☐ ULTRASOUND TO: _1.2 W/CM2 x 7 Min to cervical paraspinals B/L_
        ☐ E-STIM    TO: _X 7 min to cervical paraspinals_

B/L _____
     ☐ FLUID THERAPY    ☐ JOBST    ☐ PARAFFIN
     TO: _____
     ☐ ICE    TO: _10 min to cervical paraspinals_

B/L _____
     ☐ HOTPACKS    TO: _10 min to cervical paraspinals B/L_
     ☐ EXERCISES ☐ PROM ☐ AAROM ☐ AROM
     TO: _____
     ☒ PRE's ☐ ISOMETRICS ☐ ISOKINETICS
   TO: _B/L UE_
     ☐ SLIDEBOARD ☐ PLYOMETRICS ☐ MODIFIED KNEE BEND
☐ STEPUPS
☐ LUMBAR STABILIZATION ☐ WILLIAM's ☐ McKENZIE ☒ CERVICAL EXERCISES
☐ RELAXATION ☐ COORDINATION

MANUAL: ☐ CONTRACT RELAX ☐ CRANIOSACRAL ☐ JONES/C-STRAIN ☐ SOFT
TISSUE MOBILIZATION
     ☐ STRETCHING ☐ MASSAGE ☐ MYOF AS RELEASE ☐ SPRAY/STRETCH
   TO: _Cervical paraspinals_

EDUCATION: ☒ MOBILITY: ☐ TRANSFERS ☒ ADL ☒ HEP ☐ ENERGY CONSERV
☐ WORK HARDENING ☒ BIOMECHANICS ☐ 1
HANDED TECHNIQUES
☐ GAIT TRAINING ☐ FINE MOTOR ☐ COORD/BALANCE
OTHER: _____
_____
_____

ADL-ACTIVITIES OF DAILY LIVING    AAROM-ACTIVE/ASSISTIVERANGEOFMOTION   DBP-
DIASTOLIC BLOOD PRESSURE
SBP-SYSTOLIC BLOOD PRESSURE    HR-HEART RATE   HEP-HOME EXERCISE PROGRAM
NWB-NON-WEIGHT BEARING
PRE's-PROGRESSIVE RESISTIVE EXERCISES    WBAT-WEIGHT BEARING AS TOLERATED
ROM-RANGE OF MOTION

The above is medically necessary to decrease debility and achieve ADL independence. Also to:
☒ decrease pain, ☒ improve strength/endurance, ☒ improve balance coordination, ☐ improve gait,
☐ improve transfers,
Other _____

PHYSICIAN'S SIGNATURE _____ DATE _____

# PART 2

## SHOULDER

# CASE 5

# ROTATOR CUFF TENDONITIS

Mr. F is 28 and has had left anterior shoulder pain for 3 weeks. He is a social studies teacher in an elementary school and enjoys lifting weights. He goes to the gym five times a week but recently has developed shoulder pain when doing military press. In the last few days, he experienced a sharp twinge in his shoulder when doing overhead activities such as reaching for a glass or brushing his hair. He denies any neck pain or symptoms radiating into his arm. No numbness, tingling, or burning. He has not taken any medications for this pain. He rates the pain as 4/10 intensity at its worst (such as when doing military press) and 1/10 when at rest.

**PMHx:** None

**PSHx:** Left knee meniscus repair

**Meds:** None

**Allergies:** NKDA

**Social:** No tobacco; social EtOH

**ROS:** Noncontributory

## PHYSICAL EXAMINATION

On exam, Mr. F is a well-developed, athletic male who looks his stated age. BP: 122/70, P: 64, RR: 12. He has 5/5 strength, intact sensation, and 2+ biceps, triceps, and brachioradialis reflexes in his upper extremities bilaterally. Left glenohumeral external rotation is painful for him to perform, but he is able to do it. He has a positive Hawkin sign on the left, positive Neer's on the left, positive empty can on the left, negative

O'Brien test, apprehension test, and cross arm test. The right shoulder exam is normal. There is no scapular winging bilaterally. 2+ distal pulses are palpated bilaterally.

## Impression

Left shoulder rotator cuff impingement syndrome

**Plan**
1.  X-rays of left shoulder
2.  Physical therapy.

# PHYSICAL THERAPY

The patient is a 28-year-old male who presents with left shoulder pain that started 3 weeks ago. The pain began while lifting weights overhead, using the military press. No presentations of symptoms down the left arm.
**Scale:** 4/10 pain with overhead activities, 1/10 at rest
**Increase pain:** overhead activities; brushing hair; sleeping on the left shoulder; reaching in the cupboard.
**Decrease pain:** rest; ice

## Range of Motion

**Glenohumeral joint**
*Active*
Flexion: 130 degrees with pain
Abduction: 120 degrees with pain
IR: 35 degrees
ER: 20 degrees with pain
*Passive*
Flexion: 145 degrees
Abduction: 135 degrees with pain
IR: 40 degrees
ER: 25 degrees with pain
**Thoracic spine**
R rotation 100% limited with pectoralis
L rotation 75% limited with pectoralis
Hyperkyphosis
**Joint play**
Left GH 2/6 joint capsule
T/S T4-7 2/6
**Special tests**
Neer's +
Hawkin's +
Empty can +
Wall shoulder flexion test ꓲ (decreased T/S reversal)
**Manual muscle testing**
L teres minor 4–/5 with pain

L infraspinatus 4–/5 with pain
L supraspinatus 4–/5 with pain
B middle trapezius 4/5
**Neurodynamic assessment**
None
**Tight tender points/soft tissue restrictions**
Left upper trapezius—trigger points
Left mid trapezius—trigger points
Left teres minor/infraspinatus—trigger points
Bilateral spinalis thoracis; iliocostalis thoracis; longissumus thoracis—trigger points
Left subscapularis—myofascial adhesions
**Ergonomics**
WNL

## ASSESSMENT

The patient presents with poor glenohumeral biomechanics secondary to altered force couple relationships between the subscapularis and teres minor/infraspinatus complex. Contributing to the poor glenohumeral biomechanics is the inability for the thoracic spine to reverse itself and rotation of the thoracic spine to the left.

### Plan

Self–myofascial release/corrective flexibility/corrective exercises/corrective manual therapy/modalities

### Self–Myofascial Release

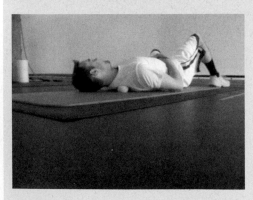

**FIGURE 5.1A.** Tennis ball roll: left posterior rotator cuff (on floor).

(*continued*)

## Self-Myofascial Release (*continued*)

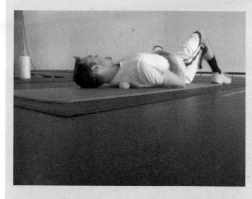

**FIGURE 5.1B.** Tennis ball roll: left middle trapezius.

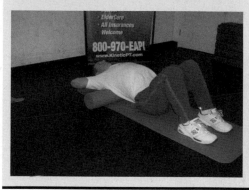

**FIGURE 5.1C.** Foam roll: T/S perpendicular.

## Corrective Flexibility

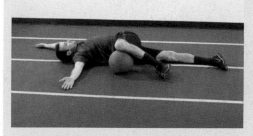

**FIGURE 5.2A.** Static: left T/S rotation/sideline/with pectoralis.

(*continued*)

## Corrective Flexibility (*continued*)

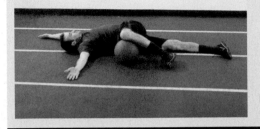

**FIGURE 5.2B.** Active: left T/S rotation/sideline/with pectoralis.

## Corrective Exercise

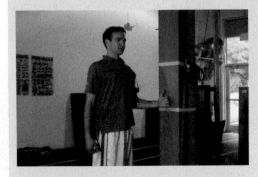

**FIGURE 5.3A.** Gradient isometric: ER 6 × 6 (gradually increase the isometric contraction).

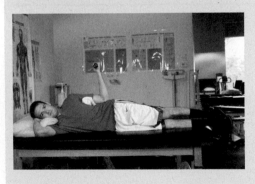

**FIGURE 5.3B.** ER: sideline/DB.

(*continued*)

## Corrective Exercise (*continued*)

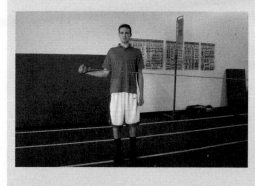

**FIGURE 5.3C.** ER: TB/parallel stance/SHARC technique (short fast external rotation).

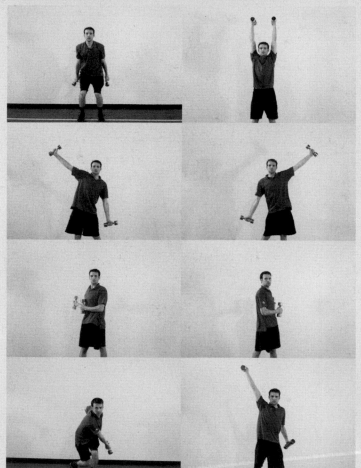

**FIGURE 5.3D.** Shoulder matrix: DB.

## Manual Therapy

1. Warming technique: left upper/mid trapezius; left posterior cuff
2. Inhibitory technique: bilateral upper trapezius/middle trapezius
3. Elongation technique: left subscapularis
4. Activating technique: left teres minor/infraspinatus/middle trapezius
5. Joint mobilization techniques: T3-6 (Grade 1–5 PA mobilization)

## Modalities: prn

1. Ice pack
2. US pulsed

## Home Exercise Program

1. Tennis ball roll: posterior rotator cuff

Orthopedic and Rehabilitation Associates
Orthopedic Street
Omaha, OH
(555) 555-5555
Fax. (666) 666-7777

PATIENT: _Mr. F_
DATE: _2009_

## ORTHOPAEDIC REHABILITATION PRESCRIPTION

*REHAB THERAPIES*    ☒ PT        ☐ OT        ☐ SESSIONS/WK _2_
TOTAL _12_

☒ NEW DIAGNOSIS    ☐ RE-EVALUATION    ☒ OUTPATIENT

DIAGNOSIS1 _Shoulder Impingement Syndrome_
    ICD _____

DIAGNOSIS2 _____
    ICD _____

PREGNANT? ☐ YES ☐ NO        PERTINENTMEDICALHISTORY: _HTN, DM_

GOALS:
MD/DO: ☒ INCREASE MOBILITY ☒ INCREASE ADL ☒ INCREASE STRENGTH ☒ DECREASE PAIN

PRECAUTIONS: ☒ CARDIAC    MAX-SBP _20_ DBP _10_ HR _20_
ABOVE BASELINE    ☒ DIABETES: HYPER/HYPOGLYCEMIA ☐ ORTHOSTASIS
☐ OTHER _____

WEIGHT BEARING:    ☐ WBAT    ☐ TIWB    ☐ NWB
    TO: _____

MODALITIES: ☐ ULTRASOUND TO: _L Shoulder x 7 Min_
            ☐ E-STIM    TO: _L Shoulder x 7 min B/L_
B/L _____
        ☐ FLUID THERAPY    ☐ JOBST    ☐ PARAFFIN
    TO: _____
        ☐ ICE    TO: _10 min to L Shoulder_
B/L _____
        ☐ HOTPACKS    TO: _10 min to L Shoulder_
        ☐ EXERCISES ☐ PROM ☐ AAROM ☐ AROM
    TO: _B/L UE_
        ☒ PRE's ☐ ISOMETRICS ☐ ISOKINETICS
    TO: _B/L UE_
        ☐ SLIDEBOARD ☐ PLYOMETRICS ☐ MODIFIED KNEE BEND
☐ STEPUPS
☐ LUMBAR STABILIZATION ☐ WILLIAM's ☐ McKENZIE ☒ CERVICAL EXERCISES
☐ RELAXATION ☐ COORDINATION
MANUAL: ☒ CONTRACT RELAX ☐ CRANIOSACRAL ☒ JONES/C-STRAIN ☒ SOFT
TISSUE MOBILIZATION
        ☒ STRETCHING ☒ MASSAGE ☒ MYOFAS RELEASE ☒ SPRAY/STRETCH
    TO: _____ UE B/L
EDUCATION: ☒ MOBILITY: ☐ TRANSFERS ☒ ADL ☒ HEP ☐ ENERGY CONSERV
    ☐ WORK HARDENING ☒ BIOMECHANICS ☐ 1
HANDED TECHNIQUES
    ☐ GAIT TRAINING ☐ FINE MOTOR ☐ COORD/BALANCE
OTHER: _____
_____
_____

ADL-ACTIVITIES OF DAILY LIVING    AAROM-ACTIVE/ASSISTIVERANGEOFMOTION    DBP-
DIASTOLIC BLOOD PRESSURE
SBP-SYSTOLIC BLOOD PRESSURE    HR-HEART RATE    HEP-HOME EXERCISE PROGRAM
NWB-NON-WEIGHT BEARING
PRE's-PROGRESSIVE RESISTIVE EXERCISES    WBAT-WEIGHT BEARING AS TOLERATED
ROM-RANGE OF MOTION

The above is medically necessary to decrease debility and achieve ADL independence. Also to:
☒ decrease pain, ☒ improve strength/endurance, ☒ improve balance coordination, ☐ improve gait,
☐ improve transfers,
Other _____

PHYSICIAN'S SIGNATURE _____    DATE _____

# CASE 6

# BICEPS TENDONITIS

**CC:** Shoulder pain

**HPI:** Mr. R is 72 years old and complains of 4 months of right shoulder pain. He says the pain began gradually and has been getting worse over the last 3 weeks. The pain is located in the anterior shoulder. He denies any neck pain or radiating symptoms. He takes Advil once in a while and this helps the symptoms. He rates the pain as 4/10 intensity.

**PMHx:** High cholesterol, HTN

**PSHx:** Prostatectomy

**Meds:** Toprol XL, HCTZ, Lipitor

**Allergies:** NKDA

**Social:** He quit smoking 10 years ago; social EtOH

**ROS:** Noncontributory

## PHYSICAL EXAMINATION

On exam, Mr. R is a well-developed male who looks his stated age. BP: 138/88, P: 60, RR: 14. He has 5/5 strength, intact sensation, and 2+ biceps, triceps, and brachioradialis reflexes in his upper extremities bilaterally. He has tenderness over the long head of the right biceps tendon as it passes through the bicipital groove of the humerus. He has a positive right Speed test, negative Hawkin, Neer, and cross arm test and a negative O'Brien test. The left shoulder exam is within normal limits.

There is no scapular winging bilaterally. 2+ distal pulses are palpated bilaterally.

## Impression

Right shoulder bicipital tendonitis

### Plan

**1.** X-rays of right shoulder
**2.** Physical therapy

# PHYSICAL THERAPY

The patient is a 72-year-old male who presents with right shoulder pain that started 4 weeks ago. The pain started from an insidious onset. Pain has progressively gotten worse over the past 3 weeks.

**Scale:** 4/10 constant ache

**Increase pain:** overhead activities; putting on seat belt; sleeping on the left shoulder; donning/doffing shirts

**Decrease pain:** meds; heat

## Range of Motion

**Glenohumeral joint**

*Active*

Flexion: 140 degrees with discomfort

Abduction: 135 degrees with discomfort

IR: 40 degrees

ER: 20 degrees with pain

*Passive*

Flexion: 150 degrees

Abduction: 145 degrees

IR: 40 degrees

ER: 25 degrees with pain

**Thoracic spine**

WNL

**Joint play**

3/6 through out

**Special tests**

Speed's +

Yergason's +

Neer's –

Hawkin's –

**Manual muscle testing**

R biceps 4/5 with pain

R infraspinatus 4/5 with pain

**Neurodynamic assessment**

None

**Tight tender points/soft tissue restrictions**
Right pectoralis major/minor—trigger points
Right biceps—trigger points
Right infraspinatus—trigger points
Right subscapularis—myofascial adhesions
Right pectoralis major and long head biceps junction—myofascial adhesion
Right latissimus dorsi—myofascial adhesions
**Ergonomics**
WNL

## ASSESSMENT

The patient presents with bicipital tendonitis that was caused by poor glenohumeral biomechanics secondary to altered force couple relationships between the subscapularis and infraspinatus. Myofascial restrictions at the junction of the long head of the biceps and the pectoralis major are limiting the efficacy of the long head to slide in the groove effectively.

### Plan

Self–myofascial release/corrective flexibility/corrective exercises/corrective manual therapy/modalities

### Self–Myofascial Release

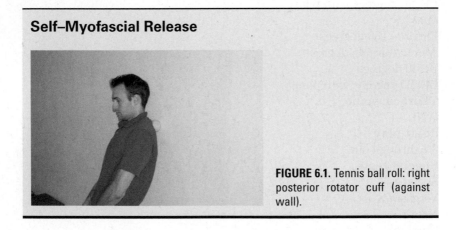

**FIGURE 6.1.** Tennis ball roll: right posterior rotator cuff (against wall).

## Corrective Flexibility

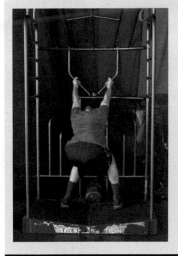

**FIGURE 6.2.** Static: right latissimus dorsi.

## Corrective Exercise

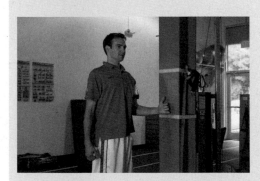

**FIGURE 6.3A.** Gradient isometric: ER 6 × 6 (gradually increase isometric contraction).

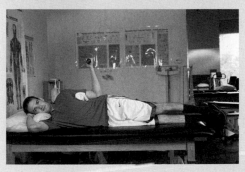

**FIGURE 6.3B.** ER: sideline/DB.

*(continued)*

## Corrective Exercise (*continued*)

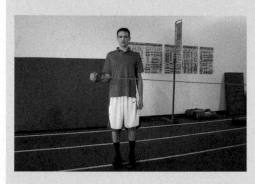

**FIGURE 6.3C.** ER: TB/parallel stance/SHARC technique (short fast ER).

(*continued*)

## Corrective Exercise (*continued*)

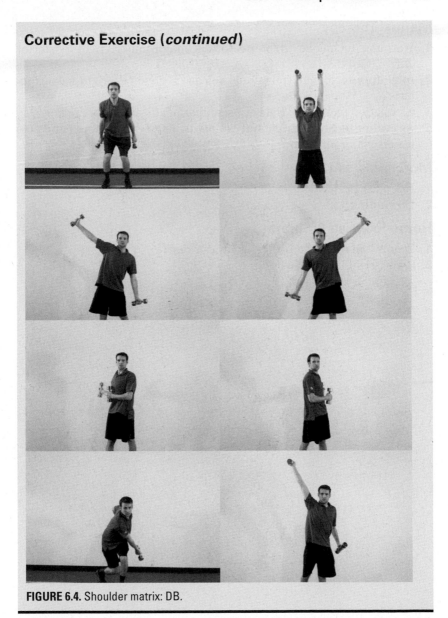

**FIGURE 6.4.** Shoulder matrix: DB.

## Manual Therapy

1. Warming technique: right pectoralis major/minor; right posterior cuff
2. Inhibitory technique (positional release technique): right subscapularis
3. Elongation technique: right subscapularis/latissimus dorsi
4. Activating technique: right infraspinatus/long head of biceps and pectoralis major junction

## Modalities: prn

1. Hot pack
2. US continuous

## Home Exercise Program

1. Tennis ball roll: right posterior rotator cuff
2. Static: right latissimus dorsi

Orthopedic and Rehabilitation Associates
Orthopedic Street
Omaha, OH
(555) 555-5555
Fax. (666) 666-7777

PATIENT: _Mr. R_
DATE: _2009_

## ORTHOPAEDIC REHABILITATION PRESCRIPTION

REHAB THERAPIES    ☒ PT    ☐ OT    ☐ SESSIONS/WK _2_
TOTAL _12_

☒ NEW DIAGNOSIS    ☐ RE-EVALUATION    ☒ OUTPATIENT

DIAGNOSIS1 _Right bicipital tendonitis_
   ICD _____

DIAGNOSIS2 _____
   ICD _____

PREGNANT? ☐ YES ☒ NO     PERTINENTMEDICALHISTORY: _HTN_

GOALS:
MD/DO: ☒ INCREASE MOBILITY ☒ INCREASE ADL ☒ INCREASE STRENGTH ☒ DECREASE PAIN

PRECAUTIONS: ☒ CARDIAC    MAX-SBP _20_ DBP _10_ HR _20_
ABOVE BASELINE    ☒ DIABETES: HYPER/HYPOGLYCEMIA ☐ ORTHOSTASIS
☐ OTHER _____

WEIGHT BEARING:    ☐ WBAT    ☐ TIWB    ☐ NWB
   TO: _____

MODALITIES: ☐ ULTRASOUND TO: _R shoulder x 1 Min_
     ☐ E-STIM    TO: _R shoulder x 1 min B/L_
B/L _____
     ☐ FLUID THERAPY    ☐ JOBST    ☐ PARAFFIN
   TO: _____
     ☐ ICE    TO: _10 min to R shoulder_
B/L _____
     ☐ HOTPACKS    TO: _10 min to R shoulder_
     ☐ EXERCISES ☐ PROM ☐ AAROM ☐ AROM
   TO: _B/L UE_
     ☒ PRE's ☐ SOMETRICS ☐ SOKINETICS
   TO: _B/L UE_
     ☐ SLIDEBOARD ☐ PLYOMETRICS ☐ MODIFIED KNEE BEND
☐ STEPUPS
☐ LUMBAR STABILIZATION ☐ WILLIAM's ☐ McKENZIE ☒ CERVICAL EXERCISES
☐ RELAXATION ☐ COORDINATION

MANUAL: ☒ CONTRACT RELAX ☐ CRANIOSACRAL ☐ JONES/C-STRAIN ☐ SOFT
TISSUE MOBILIZATION
     ☐ STRETCHING ☐ MASSAGE ☐ MYOF AS RELEASE ☐ SPRAY/STRETCH
   TO: _____ Cervicalparaspinals
EDUCATION: ☒ MOBILITY: ☐ TRANSFERS ☒ ADL ☒ HEP ☐ ENERGY CONSERV
☐ WORK HARDENING ☒ BIOMECHANICS ☐ 1
HANDED TECHNIQUES
☐ GAIT TRAINING ☐ FINE MOTOR ☐ COORD/BALANCE
OTHER: _____
_____
_____

ADL-ACTIVITIES OF DAILY LIVING    AAROM-ACTIVE/ASSISTIVERANGEOFMOTION   DBP-
DIASTOLIC BLOOD PRESSURE
SBP-SYSTOLIC BLOOD PRESSURE    HR-HEART RATE    HEP-HOME EXERCISE PROGRAM
NWB-NON-WEIGHT BEARING
PRE's-PROGRESSIVE RESISTIVE EXERCISES    WBAT-WEIGHT BEARING AS TOLERATED
ROM-RANGE OF MOTION

The above is medically necessary to decrease debility and achieve ADL independence. Also to:
☒ decrease pain, ☒ improve strength/endurance, ☒ improve balance coordination, ☐ improve gait,
☐ improve transfers,
Other _____

PHYSICIAN'S SIGNATURE _____ DATE _____

# CASE 7

# LEFT AC JOINT ARTHRITIS

**CC:** Left shoulder pain

**HPI:** Mr. Z is 43 years old and complains of left shoulder pain. The pain is a dull ache and has been present for about 2 months. It began gradually and has gotten worse. When Mr. Z points to the pain, he points to his AC joint. The pain is worse with carrying heavy loads and doing the bench press in the gym. On average, VAS = 4/10. He denies any numbness, tingling, burning, or weakness. He denies any neck pain or radiating symptoms. He cannot remember having pain like this before, but he does note that he played football in college and was "always getting hurt." He never fractured his collar bone. He takes over-the-counter NSAIDs before going to the gym and says this helps him do his workout with less pain.

**PMHx:** None
**PSHx:** Tonsillectomy
**Meds:** Advil prn
**Allergies:** NKDA
**Social:** No tobacco; social EtOH
**ROS:** Noncontributory

## PHYSICAL EXAMINATION

On exam, Mr. Z is a well-developed, athletic male who looks his stated age. BP: 122/70, P: 64, RR: 12. He has 5/5 strength, intact sensation, and 2+ biceps, triceps, and brachioradialis reflexes in his upper extremities bilaterally. Left glenohumeral external rotation is painful for him to perform, but he is able to do it. He has a positive Hawkin sign on the left, positive Neer on the left, positive empty can on the left, negative O'Brien test, apprehension test, and cross arm test. The right shoulder exam is normal. There is no scapular winging bilaterally. 2+ distal pulses are palpated bilaterally.

## Impression

Left AC joint arthritis

## Plan

1. X-rays of left shoulder
2. Physical therapy

# PHYSICAL THERAPY

The patient is a 43-year-old male who presents with left shoulder pain that started 2 weeks ago. The pain has gradually gotten worse and went to his medical doctor. The patient was diagnosed with AC joint arthritis and his physician recommended physical therapy. The patient has a history of trauma to his left shoulder while playing football in college.

**Scale:** 6–8/10 pain at most and 2/10 at rest

**Increase pain:** lifting heavy loads; bench pressing; putting on his seat belt

**Decrease pain:** meds; heat

## Range of Motion

**Glenohumeral joint**

*Active*

Flexion: 140 degrees with discomfort
Abduction: 135 degrees with discomfort
IR: 40 degrees
ER: 20 degrees with pain

*Passive*

Flexion: 150 degrees
Abduction: 145 degrees
IR: 40 degrees
ER: 25 degrees with pain

**Thoracic spine**

WNL

**Joint play**

3/6 through out

**Special tests**

Speed's +
Yergason's +
Neer's –
Hawkin's –

**Manual muscle testing**
R biceps 4/5 with pain
R infraspinatus 4/5 with pain
**Neurodynamic assessment**
None
**Tight tender points/soft tissue restrictions**
Right pectoralis major/minor—trigger points
Right biceps—trigger points
Right infraspinatus—trigger points
Right subscapularis—myofascial adhesions
Right pectoralis major and long head biceps junction—myofascial adhesion
Right latissimus dorsi—myofascial adhesions
**Ergonomics**
WNL

## ASSESSMENT

The patient presents with bicipital tendonitis that was caused by poor glenohumeral biomechanics secondary to altered force couple relationships between the subscapularis and infraspinatus. Myofascial restrictions at the junction of the long head of the biceps and the pectoralis major are limiting the efficacy of the long head to slide in the groove effectively.

### Plan

Self–myofascial release/corrective flexibility/corrective exercises/corrective manual therapy/modalities

---

**Self–Myofascial Release**

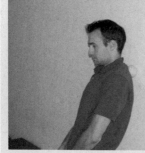

**FIGURE 7.1.** Tennis ball roll: right posterior rotator cuff (against wall).

## Corrective Flexibility

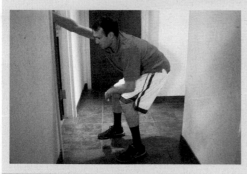

**FIGURE 7.2.** Static: right latissimus dorsi.

## Corrective Exercise

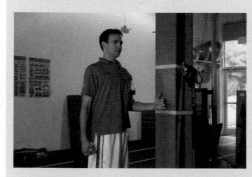

**FIGURE 7.3A.** Gradient isometric: ER 6 × 6 (gradually increase isometric contraction).

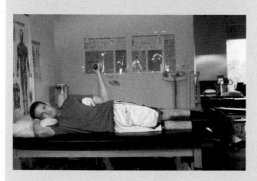

**FIGURE 7.3B.** ER: sideline/DB.

*(continued)*

## Corrective Exercise (*continued*)

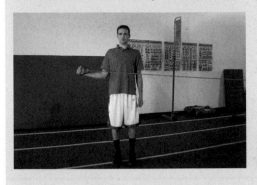

**FIGURE 7.3C.** ER: TB/parallel stance/SHARC technique (short fast ER).

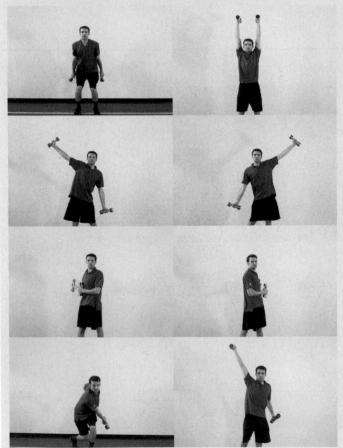

**FIGURE 7.3D.** Shoulder matrix: DB.

## Manual Therapy

1. Warming technique: right pectoralis major/minor; right posterior cuff
2. Inhibitory technique: right subscapularis
3. Elongation technique: right subscapularis/latissimus dorsi
4. Activating technique: right infraspinatus/long head of biceps and pectoralis major junction

## Modalities: prn

1. Hot pack
2. US continuous

## Home Exercise Program

1. Tennis ball roll: right posterior rotator cuff
2. Static: right latissimus dorsi

Orthopedic and Rehabilitation Associates
Orthopedic Street
Omaha, OH
(555) 555-5555
Fax. (666) 666-7777

PATIENT: _Mr. Z_
DATE: _2009_

## ORTHOPAEDIC REHABILITATION PRESCRIPTION

| REHAB THERAPIES | ☒ PT | ☐ OT | ☐ SESSIONS/WK _2_ |

TOTAL _12_

☒ NEW DIAGNOSIS   ☐ RE-EVALUATION   ☒ OUTPATIENT

DIAGNOSIS1 _AC joint arthritis_
  ICD _____

DIAGNOSIS2 _____
  ICD _____

PREGNANT? ☐ YES ☒ NO       PERTINENTMEDICALHISTORY: _None_

GOALS:
MD/DO: ☒ INCREASE MOBILITY ☒ INCREASE ADL ☒ INCREASE STRENGTH ☒ DECREASE PAIN

PRECAUTIONS: ☒ CARDIAC     MAX-SBP_____ DBP_____ HR_____
ABOVE BASELINE     ☒ DIABETES: HYPER/HYPOGLYCEMIA ☐ ORTHOSTASIS
  ☐ OTHER _____
WEIGHT BEARING:   ☐ WBAT   ☐ TTWB   ☐ NWB
  TO: _____
MODALITIES: ☐ ULTRASOUND TO: _L shoulder x 7 min_
          ☐ E-STIM     TO: _L shoulder x 7 min B/L_
B/L _____
      ☐ FLUID THERAPY   ☐ JOBST   ☐ PARAFFIN
  TO: _____
      ☐ ICE   TO: _10 min to L shoulder_
B/L _____
      ☐ HOTPACKS   TO: _10 min to L shoulder_
      ☐ EXERCISES ☐ PROM ☐ AAROM ☐ AROM
  TO: _B/L UE_
      ☒ PRE's ☐ ISOMETRICS ☐ ISOKINETICS
  TO: _B/L UE_
      ☐ SLIDEBOARD ☐ PLYOMETRICS ☐ MODIFIED KNEE BEND
☐ STEPUPS
☐ LUMBAR STABILIZATION ☐ WILLIAM's ☐ McKENZIE ☒ CERVICAL EXERCISES
☐ RELAXATION ☐ COORDINATION
MANUAL: ☒ CONTRACT RELAX ☐ CRANIOSACRAL ☒ JONES/C-STRAIN ☒ SOFT
TISSUE MOBILIZATION
      ☒ STRETCHING ☒ MASSAGE ☒ MYOF AS RELEASE ☒ SPRAY/STRETCH
  TO: _UE B/L_
EDUCATION: ☒ MOBILITY: ☐ TRANSFERS ☒ ADL ☒ HEP ☐ ENERGY CONSERV
  ☐ WORK HARDENING ☒ BIOMECHANICS ☐ 1
HANDED TECHNIQUES
  ☐ GAIT TRAINING ☐ FINE MOTOR ☐ COORD/BALANCE
OTHER: _____
_____
_____

ADL-ACTIVITIES OF DAILY LIVING     AAROM-ACTIVE/ASSISTIVERANGEOFMOTION   DBP-
DIASTOLIC BLOOD PRESSURE
SBP-SYSTOLIC BLOOD PRESSURE   HR-HEART RATE   HEP-HOME EXERCISE PROGRAM
NWB-NON-WEIGHT BEARING
PRE's-PROGRESSIVE RESISTIVE EXERCISES   WBAT-WEIGHT BEARING AS TOLERATED
ROM-RANGE OF MOTION

The above is medically necessary to decrease debility and achieve ADL independence. Also to:
☒ decrease pain, ☒ improve strength/endurance, ☒ improve balance coordination, ☐ improve gait,
☐ improve transfers,
Other _____

PHYSICIAN'S SIGNATURE _____ DATE _____

# CASE 8

# LABRAL TEAR

**CC:** Right shoulder pain

**HPI:** Ms. M is 40 years old and has had shoulder pain for over 6 months. She says the pain began when she fell onto an out-stretched arm (after slipping on ice). She never had it looked at by a doctor, but the pain just got better over the course of several weeks. However, it never got completely better and she continues to have a dull ache in the entire right shoulder. She rates the pain as 3/10 intensity. The pain is worse with activities that require any force with her arm (such as shoveling snow and picking up her 7-year-old daughter). She denies any numbness, tingling, or burning. She does not describe any neck pain or radiating symptoms. She does not take any medications for pain.

**PMHx:** None

**PSHx:** None

**Meds:** None

**Allergies:** NKDA

**Social:** No tobacco; no EtOH

**ROS:** Noncontributory

## PHYSICAL EXAMINATION

On exam, Ms. M is a well-developed female who looks her stated age. BP: 116/80, P: 74, RR: 14. She has 5/5 strength, intact sensation, and 2+ biceps, triceps, and brachioradialis reflexes in her upper extremities bilaterally. Right O'Brien test is positive. Otherwise, she has a negative apprehension test, negative Hawkin, Neer, empty can test, and Speed test on the right. The left shoulder exam is within normal limits. There is no scapular winging bilaterally. 2+ distal pulses are palpated bilaterally.

## Impression

Right glenoid labral tear

**Plan**

1. X-rays of right shoulder
2. Physical therapy

# PHYSICAL THERAPY

The patient is a 40-year-old female who presents with right shoulder pain that started 6 months ago after slipping on ice and landing on her out-stretched arm. The pain has progressively gotten worse and the patient went to her physician to get it looked at. The pain is a deep dull ache.

**Scale:** 3/10 pain

**Increase pain:** lifting loads >15 lb; carrying groceries; pushing shopping cart; carrying her daughter; shoveling snow

**Decrease pain:** nothing

## Range of Motion

**Glenohumeral joint**

*Active*

Flexion: 160 degrees with discomfort

Abduction: 150 degrees with discomfort

IR: WNL

ER: WNL with dull ache

*Passive*

Flexion: 160 degrees

Abduction: 150 degrees

IR: WNL

ER: WNL with dull ache at end range

**Thoracic spine**

WNL

**Joint play**

Anterior: empty end feel

**Special tests**

O'Brien's +

Empty can −

Neer's −

Hawkin's −

**Manual muscle testing**

R teres minor 4/5

R infraspinatus 4/5

R subscapularis 4/5
R pectoralis major clavicular portion 4/5
**Neurodynamic assessment**
None
**Tight tender points/soft tissue restrictions**
Right pectoralis major/minor—trigger points
Right subclavius—trigger points
Right infraspinatus—trigger points
Right teres minor—trigger points
**Ergonomics**
WNL

## ASSESSMENT

The patient presents with right labral tear with weakness of periglenohumeral joint muscles, including teres minor; infraspinatus; subscapularis; and clavicular portion of the pectoralis major. Trigger points noted at right subclavius, infraspinatus; teres minor; and pectoralis major and minor. Joint play of the right anterior joint capsule is empty, with noticeable joint capsular instability.

### Plan

Self–myofascial release/corrective flexibility/corrective exercises/corrective manual therapy/modalities

---

### Self–Myofascial Release

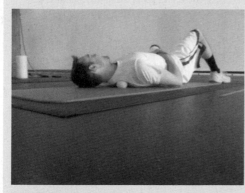

**FIGURE 8.1.** Tennis ball roll: right posterior rotator cuff (floor).

## Corrective Flexibility

1. None

## Corrective Exercise

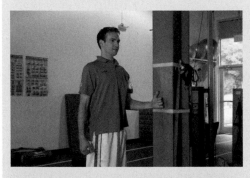

**FIGURE 8.2A.** Gradient isometric: ER 6 × 6 (gradually increase isometric contraction).

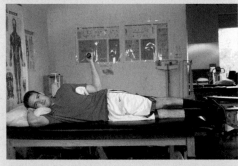

**FIGURE 8.2B.** ER: sideline/DB.

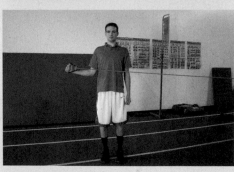

**FIGURE 8.2C.** ER: TB/parallel stance/SHARC technique (short fast ER).

(*continued*)

## Corrective Exercise (*continued*)

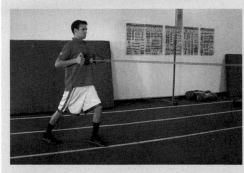

**FIGURE 8.2D.** Pull: split stance/ theraband/two arms.

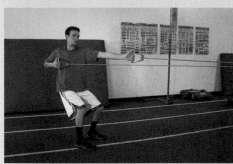

**FIGURE 8.2E.** Pull: parallel stance/ theraband/total body rotation.

## Manual Therapy

1. Warming technique: right pectoralis major/minor; right posterior cuff
2. Inhibitory technique: right subscapularis
3. Activating technique: right infraspinatus/teres minor/clavicular portion of the pectoralis major

## Modalities: prn

1. NA

## Home Exercise Program

1. Tennis ball roll: right posterior rotator cuff
2. Gradient isometric: ER 6 × 6

Orthopedic and Rehabilitation Associates
Orthopedic Street
Omaha, OH
(555) 555-5555
Fax. (666) 666-7777

PATIENT: _Ms, M_
DATE: _2009_

## ORTHOPAEDIC REHABILITATION PRESCRIPTION

| REHAB THERAPIES | ☒ PT | ☐ OT | ☐ SESSIONS/WK _2_ |
|---|---|---|---|

TOTAL _12_

☒ NEW DIAGNOSIS    ☐ RE-EVALUATION    ☒ OUTPATIENT

DIAGNOSIS1 _Glenoid labral tear_
   ICD _____

DIAGNOSIS2 _____
   ICD _____

PREGNANT? ☐ YES ☒ NO     PERTINENTMEDICALHISTORY: _None_

GOALS:
MD/DO: ☒ INCREASE MOBILITY ☒ INCREASE ADL ☒ INCREASE STRENGTH ☒ DECREASE PAIN

PRECAUTIONS: ☐ CARDIAC    MAX-SBP____ DBP____ HR____
ABOVE BASELINE  ☐ DIABETES: HYPER/HYPOGLYCEMIA ☐ ORTHOSTASIS
☐ OTHER _____
WEIGHT BEARING:  ☐ WBAT  ☐ TTWB  ☐ NWB
   TO: _____
MODALITIES: ☐ ULTRASOUND TO: _R shoulder x 7 min_
       ☐ E-STIM    TO: _R shoulder x 7 B/L_
B/L _____
      ☐ FLUID THERAPY    ☐ JOBST    ☐ PARAFFIN
   TO: _____
      ☐ ICE    TO: _10 min to R shoulder_
B/L _____
      ☐ HOTPACKS    TO: _10 min to R shoulder_
      ☐ EXERCISES ☐ PROM ☐ AAROM ☐ AROM
   TO: B/L UE _____
      ☒ PRE's ☐ ISOMETRICS ☐ ISOKINETICS
   TO: _B/L UE_ _____
      ☐ SLIDEBOARD ☐ PLYOMETRICS ☐ MODIFIED KNEE BEND
☐ STEPUPS
☐ LUMBAR STABILIZATION ☐ WILLIAM's ☐ McKENZIE ☒ CERVICAL EXERCISES
☐ RELAXATION ☐ COORDINATION
MANUAL: ☒ CONTRACT RELAX ☐ CRANIOSACRAL ☒ JONES/C-STRAIN ☒ SOFT
TISSUE MOBILIZATION
      ☒ STRETCHING ☒ MASSAGE ☒ MYOF AS RELEASE ☐ SPRAY/STRETCH
   TO: _UE B/L_ _____
EDUCATION: ☒ MOBILITY: ☐ TRANSFERS ☒ ADL ☒ HEP ☐ ENERGY CONSERV
   ☐ WORK HARDENING ☒ BIOMECHANICS ☐ 1
HANDED TECHNIQUES
   ☐ GAIT TRAINING ☐ FINE MOTOR ☐ COORD/BALANCE
OTHER: _____
_____
_____

ADL-ACTIVITIES OF DAILY LIVING    AAROM-ACTIVE/ASSISTIVERANGEOFMOTION   DBP-
DIASTOLIC BLOOD PRESSURE
SBP-SYSTOLIC BLOOD PRESSURE    HR-HEART RATE    HEP-HOME EXERCISE PROGRAM
NWB-NON-WEIGHT BEARING
PRE's-PROGRESSIVE RESISTIVE EXERCISES    WBAT-WEIGHT BEARING AS TOLERATED
ROM-RANGE OF MOTION

The above is medically necessary to decrease debility and achieve ADL independence. Also to:
☒ decrease pain, ☒ improve strength/endurance, ☒ improve balance coordination, ☐ improve gait,
☐ improve transfers,
Other _____

PHYSICIAN'S SIGNATURE _____ DATE _____

# PART 3

## ELBOW

# CASE 9

## LATERAL EPICONDYLITIS

**CC:** Right elbow pain

**HPI:** Mr. B is a 33-year-old male with right elbow pain for the last 2 weeks. He says it began while he was putting together his son's new baby crib and has gotten worse since then. The pain is on the lateral aspect of the elbow. He denies any numbness, tingling, or burning sensation. The pain is worse when using his right upper extremity, such as when shaking hands, throwing a ball or anything else that requires force with his hand. He has not taken any pain medications. On a scale of 0 to 10, he rates the pain, on average, a 4/10.

**PMHx:** None

**PSHx:** None

**Meds:** None

**Allergies:** NKDA

**Social:** No tobacco. Social EtOH

**ROS:** Noncontributory

## PHYSICAL EXAMINATION

On exam, Mr. B is a well-developed male who looks his stated age. BP: 124/78, P: 62, RR: 14. He has 5/5 strength, intact sensation, and 2+ biceps, triceps, and brachioradialis reflexes in his upper extremities bilaterally. He has tenderness over the lateral aspect of the right elbow. He has a positive Cozen, Maudsley, and Mill tests on the right. Examination of his left elbow is within normal limits. 2+ distal pulses are palpated bilaterally.

## Impression
Right lateral epicondylitis

**Plan**
**1.** Physical therapy

# PHYSICAL THERAPY

The patient is a 33-year-old male who presents with right elbow pain that started 2 weeks ago while putting together his son's new baby crib. Pain has been progressing and recently, the patient went to his physician who referred the patient to physical therapy.

**Scale:** 4/10 pain
**Increase pain:** lifting loads >10 lb; shaking hands; pouring a glass of milk; carrying anything >10 lb
**Decrease pain:** rest

## Range of Motion

**Wrist**
Wrist flexion: WNL with lateral elbow discomfort
Wrist extension: WNL
Radial deviation: WNL
Ulna deviation: WNL
Supination: 30 degrees
Pronation: WNL

**Elbow**
Flexion: WNL
Extension: –5 degrees

**Shoulder**
Flexion: 140 degrees

**Joint play**
WNL

**Special tests**
Cozen's +
Maudsley +
Mill's +

**Manual muscle testing**
R brachioradialis 4/5 with pain
R extensor carpi radialis longus 4/5 with pain

**Neurodynamic assessment**
Radial nerve

**Tight tender points/soft tissue restrictions**
Right pectoralis minor—trigger points
Right subclavius—trigger points
Right brachioradialis—trigger points
Right extensor carpi radialis longus—trigger points
Right pronator teres—myofascial restrictions
Right latissimus dorsi—myofascial restrictions

**Ergonomics**
WNL

## ASSESSMENT

The patient presents with right elbow pain that is indicative of lateral epicondylitis. Muscle weakness of the brachioradialis and extensor carpi radialis longus along with decreased supination from myofascial restrictions noted in the pronator teres are contributing factors to the patient's pain. Both trigger points noted in the pectoralis major and sub-clavius refer into the right elbow.

### Plan

Self–myofascial release/corrective flexibility/corrective exercises/corrective manual therapy/modalities

---

### Self Myofascial Release

1. None

---

### Corrective Flexibility

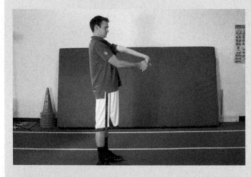

**FIGURE 9.1A.** Static: wrist flexion.

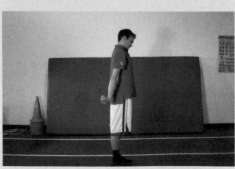

**FIGURE 9.1B.** Neurodynamic: radial nerve stretch.

## Corrective Exercise

1. Phase 1: Pain Management Phase—Exercise should be limited secondary to the repetitive trauma of the elbow for the first 2 weeks until pain is resolved.
2. Phase 2: Exercise is slowly introduced.

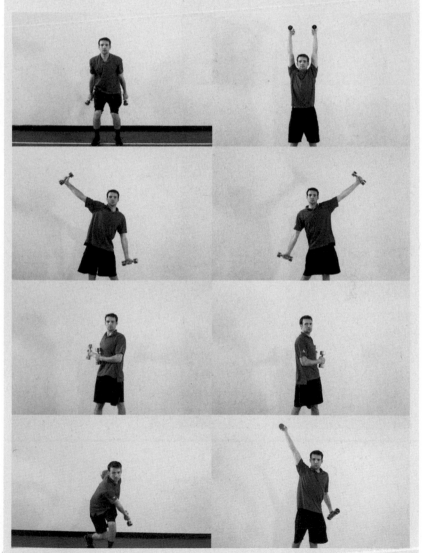

**FIGURE 9.2A.** Shoulder matrix.

(*continued*)

## Corrective Exercise (*continued*)

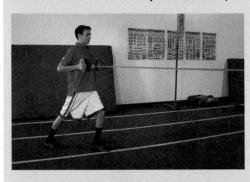

**FIGURE 9.2B.** Pull: split stance/ theraband/two arms.

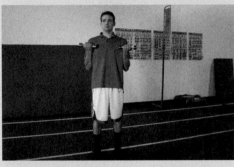

**FIGURE 9.2C.** Bicep curls: palm up.

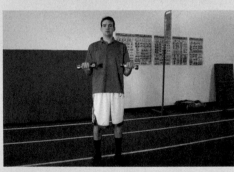

**FIGURE 9.2D.** Bicep curls: palm down.

## Manual Therapy

1. Warming technique: brachioradialis; extensor carpi radialis longus; anconeus
2. Inhibitory technique: right brachioradialis; subclavius; pectoralis minor
3. Activation technique: right brachioradialis; extensor carpi radialis longus/brevis
4. Elongation technique: pronator teres

## Modalities: prn

1. Ice pack
2. US pulse

## Home Exercise Program

1. Neurodynamic: radial nerve
2. Ice

Orthopedic and Rehabilitation Associates
Orthopedic Street
Omaha, OH
(555) 555-5555
Fax. (666) 666-7777

PATIENT: _Mr. B_
DATE: _2009_

## ORTHOPAEDIC REHABILITATION PRESCRIPTION

| _REHAB THERAPIES_ | ☒ PT | ☐ OT | ☐ SESSIONS/WK _2_ |
| --- | --- | --- | --- |
| TOTAL _12_ | | | |

☒ NEW DIAGNOSIS    ☐ RE-EVALUATION    ☒ OUTPATIENT

DIAGNOSIS1 _Lateral epicondylitis_
   ICD _____

DIAGNOSIS2 _____
   ICD _____

PREGNANT? ☐ YES ☒ NO     PERTINENTMEDICALHISTORY: _None_

GOALS:
MD/DO: ☒ INCREASE MOBILITY ☒ INCREASE ADL ☒ INCREASE STRENGTH ☒ DECREASE PAIN

PRECAUTIONS: ☐ CARDIAC    MAX-SBP _____ DBP _____ HR _____
ABOVE BASELINE   ☐ DIABETES: HYPER/HYPOGLYCEMIA ☐ ORTHOSTASIS
☐ OTHER _____
WEIGHT BEARING:   ☐ WBAT   ☐ TTWB   ☐ NWB
   TO: _____
MODALITIES: ☐ ULTRASOUND TO: _R elbow x 1 min_
      ☐ E-STIM    TO: _R elbow x 1 min B/L_
B/L _____
    ☐ FLUID THERAPY    ☐ JOBST    ☐ PARAFFIN
   TO: _____
    ☐ ICE    TO: _10 min to R elbow_
B/L _____
    ☐ HOTPACKS    TO: _10 min to R elbow_
    ☐ EXERCISES ☐ PROM ☐ AAROM ☐ AROM
   TO: _B/L UE_
    ☒ PRE's ☐ ISOMETRICS ☐ ISOKINETICS
   TO: _B/L UE_
    ☐ SLIDEBOARD ☐ PLYOMETRICS ☐ MODIFIED KNEE BEND
☐ STEPUPS
☐ LUMBAR STABILIZATION ☐ WILLIAM's ☐ McKENZIE ☒ CERVICAL EXERCISES
☐ RELAXATION ☐ COORDINATION
MANUAL: ☒ CONTRACT RELAX ☐ CRANIOSACRAL ☒ JONES/C-STRAIN ☒ SOFT
TISSUE MOBILIZATION
    ☒ STRETCHING ☒ MASSAGE ☒ MYOF AS RELEASE ☒ SPRAY/STRETCH
   TO: _UE B/L_
EDUCATION: ☒ MOBILITY: ☐ TRANSFERS ☒ ADL ☒ HEP ☐ ENERGY CONSERV
☐ WORK HARDENING ☒ BIOMECHANICS ☐ 1
HANDED TECHNIQUES
☐ GAIT TRAINING ☐ FINE MOTOR ☐ COORD/BALANCE
OTHER: _____
_____
_____

ADL-ACTIVITIES OF DAILY LIVING    AAROM-ACTIVE/ASSISTIVERANGEOFMOTION    DBP-
DIASTOLIC BLOOD PRESSURE
SBP-SYSTOLIC BLOOD PRESSURE    HR-HEART RATE    HEP-HOME EXERCISE PROGRAM
NWB-NON-WEIGHT BEARING
PRE's-PROGRESSIVE RESISTIVE EXERCISES    WBAT-WEIGHT BEARING AS TOLERATED
ROM-RANGE OF MOTION

The above is medically necessary to decrease debility and achieve ADL independence. Also to:
☒ decrease pain, ☒ improve strength/endurance, ☒ improve balance coordination, ☐ improve gait,
☐ improve transfers,
Other _____

PHYSICIAN'S SIGNATURE _____ DATE _____

# CASE **10**

## MEDIAL EPICONDYLITIS

**CC:** Right elbow pain

**HPI:** Mr. Q is 46 years old and presents with 2 weeks of right medial elbow pain. He works as a plumber and first noticed the pain while at work. Since then, the pain has gotten worse. It does not radiate. He denies any numbness, tingling, or burning. Over the last 2 days, he says that even shaking hands has become painful. He does not take any medications for the pain. The pain is rated as 5/10. This is the first time he is coming to the doctor for this problem.

**PMHx:** None

**PSHx:** None

**Meds:** None

**Allergies:** NKDA

**Social:** No tobacco; social EtOH

**ROS:** Noncontributory

## PHYSICAL EXAMINATION

On exam, Mr. Q is a well-developed male who looks his stated age. BP: 130/80, P: 60, RR: 14. He has 5/5 strength, intact sensation, and 2+ biceps, triceps, and brachioradialis reflexes in his upper extremities bilaterally. He has tenderness over the medial aspect of the right elbow. Pain is reproduced with resisted wrist flexion. Examination of his left elbow is within normal limits. 2+ distal pulses are palpated bilaterally.

## Impression

Right medial epicondylitis

**Plan**

**1.** Physical therapy

# PHYSICAL THERAPY

The patient is a 46-year-old male who presents with right medial elbow pain that started 2 weeks ago while working as a plumber. Pain has been progressing and recently the patient went to his physician who referred the patient to physical therapy.

**Scale:** 5/10 pain

**Increase pain:** lifting loads >15 lb; shaking hands; pouring a glass of milk; carrying anything >10 lb; using a hammer

**Decrease pain:** rest

## Range of Motion

**Wrist**

Wrist flexion: WNL

Wrist extension: WNL with lateral elbow discomfort

Radial deviation: WNL

Ulna deviation: WNL

Supination: 35 degrees

Pronation: WNL

**Elbow**

Flexion: WNL

Extension: –5 degrees

**Shoulder**

WNL

**Joint play**

WNL

**Manual muscle testing**

R flexor carpi ulnaris 4/5 with pain

**Neurodynamic assessment**

Ulnar nerve

**Tight tender points/soft tissue restrictions**

Right biceps brachii—trigger points

Right brachioradialis—trigger points

Right pronator teres—myofascial restrictions

Right flexor carpi ulnaris—myofascial restrictions

Right medial intermuscular septum—myofascial restrictions

**Ergonomics**

WNL

## ASSESSMENT

The patient presents with right medial elbow pain that is indicative of medial epicondylitis. Muscle weakness and trigger points of the flexor carpi ulnaris, trigger points located in the brachioradialis and biceps, and myofascial restrictions noted in the pronator teres and intermuscular septum are contributing factors of the patient's pain.

### Plan

Self–myofascial release/corrective flexibility/corrective exercises/corrective manual therapy/modalities

---

### Self–Myofascial Release

1. None

---

### Corrective Flexibility

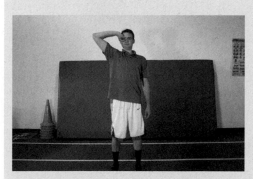

FIGURE 10.1. Neurodynamic: ulnar nerve.

---

### Corrective Exercise

1. Phase 1: Pain management phase—exercise should be limited secondary to the repetitive trauma of the elbow for the first 2 weeks until pain is resolved.
2. Phase 2: Exercise is slowly introduced.

(*continued*)

## Corrective Exercise (*continued*)

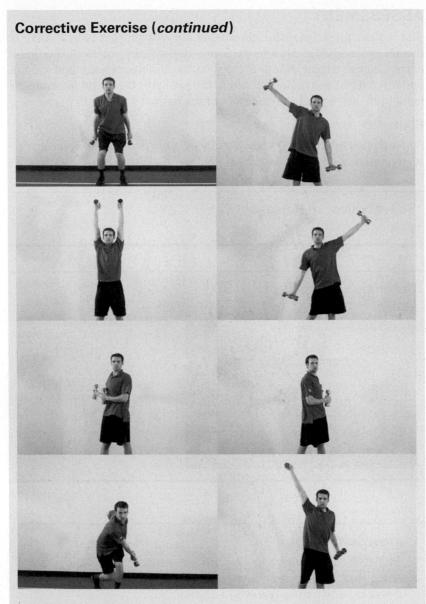

**FIGURE 10.2A.** Shoulder matrix.

(*continued*)

## Corrective Exercise (*continued*)

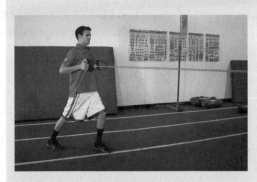

**FIGURE 10.2B.** Pull: split stance/theraband/two arms.

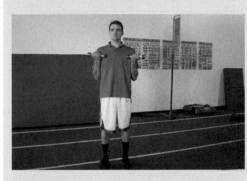

**FIGURE 10.2C.** Bicep curls: palm up.

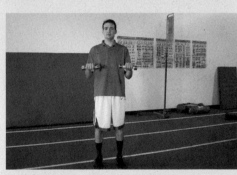

**FIGURE 10.2D.** Bicep curls: palm down.

## Manual Therapy

1. Warming technique: brachioradialis; flexor carpi ulnaris; wrist flexors; medial intermuscular septum; biceps brachii
2. Inhibitory technique: right brachioradialis; flexor carpi ulnaris; biceps brachii
3. Activation technique: right brachioradialis; flexor carpi ulnaris
4. Elongation technique: pronator teres; flexor carpi ulnaris; biceps brachii

## Modalities: prn

1. Ice pack
2. US pulse

## Home Exercise Program

1. Neurodynamic: ulnar nerve
2. Ice pack

Orthopedic and Rehabilitation Associates
Orthopedic Street
Omaha, OH
(555) 555-5555
Fax. (666) 666-7777

PATIENT: *Mr. Q*
DATE: *2009*

## ORTHOPAEDIC REHABILITATION PRESCRIPTION

*REHAB THERAPIES* ☒ PT ☐ OT ☐ SESSIONS/WK *2*
TOTAL *12*

☒ NEW DIAGNOSIS ☐ RE-EVALUATION ☒ OUTPATIENT

DIAGNOSIS1 *Medial epicondylitis*
    ICD _____

DIAGNOSIS2 _____
    ICD _____

PREGNANT? ☐ YES ☒ NO     PERTINENTMEDICALHISTORY: *None*

GOALS:
MD/DO: ☒ INCREASE MOBILITY ☒ INCREASE ADL ☒ INCREASE STRENGTH ☒ DECREASE PAIN

PRECAUTIONS: ☐ CARDIAC    MAX-SBP_____ DBP_____ HR_____
ABOVE BASELINE    ☐ DIABETES: HYPER/HYPOGLYCEMIA ☐ ORTHOSTASIS
☐ OTHER _____

WEIGHT BEARING:    ☐ WBAT    ☐ TTWB    ☐ NWB
    TO: _____

MODALITIES: ☐ ULTRASOUND TO: *R elbow x 1 Min*
            ☐ E-STIM    TO: *R elbow x 1 B/L*
B/L _____

        ☐ FLUID THERAPY    ☐ JOBST    ☐ PARAFFIN
    TO: _____
        ☐ ICE    TO: *10 min to R elbow*
B/L _____

        ☐ HOTPACKS    TO: *10 min to cervical paraspinals B/L*
        ☐ EXERCISES ☐ PROM ☐ AAROM ☐ AROM
    TO: _____
        ☐ XPRE's ☐ ISOMETRICS ☐ ISOKINETICS
    TO: _____
        ☐ SLIDEBOARD ☐ PLYOMETRICS ☐ MODIFIED KNEE BEND
☐ STEPUPS
☐ LUMBAR STABILIZATION ☐ WILLIAM's ☐ McKENZIE ☒ CERVICAL EXERCISES
☐ RELAXATION ☐ COORDINATION

MANUAL: ☒ CONTRACT RELAX ☐ CRANIOSACRAL ☒ JONES/C-STRAIN ☒ SOFT
TISSUE MOBILIZATION
        ☒ STRETCHING ☒ MASSAGE ☒ MYOF AS RELEASE ☒ SPRAY/STRETCH
    TO: *UE B/L*

EDUCATION: ☐ MOBILITY: ☐ TRANSFERS ☐ ADL ☐ HEP ☐ ENERGY CONSERV
    ☐ WORK HARDENING ☒ BIOMECHANICS ☐ 1
HANDED TECHNIQUES
☐ GAIT TRAINING ☐ FINE MOTOR ☐ COORD/BALANCE
OTHER: _____
_____

The above is medically necessary to decrease debility and achieve ADL independence. Also to:
☐ decrease pain, ☐ improve strength/endurance, ☐ improve balance coordination, ☐ improve gait,
☐ improve transfers,
Other _____

PHYSICIAN'S SIGNATURE _____    DATE _____

# PART **4**

## WRIST AND HAND

# CASE 11

# CARPAL TUNNEL SYNDROME

**CC:** Hand numbness and tingling

**HPI:** Ms. G is a 34-year-old right-handed administrative assistant who complains of numbness and tingling in her right hand, digits one through three. The symptoms are worse when typing at a computer, and sometimes she wakes up at night, at which point she shakes her hand and it feels better. The symptoms have been present, off and on, for 3 months, but have gotten worse in the last month. No neck or arm pain. No weakness.

**PMHx:** None

**PSHx:** None

**Meds:** None

**Allergies:** NKDA

**Social:** No tobacco; social EtOH

**ROS:** Noncontributory

## PHYSICAL EXAMINATION

On exam, Ms. G is a well-developed female who looks her stated age. BP: 110/70, P: 60, RR: 14. She has 5/5 strength, intact sensation, and 2+ biceps, triceps, and brachioradialis reflexes in her upper extremities bilaterally. She has a positive Phalen test that reproduces her right hand symptoms. She has a positive right carpal compression and Tinel test, both reproducing her symptoms. 2+ distal pulses are palpated bilaterally.

## Impression

Right carpal tunnel syndrome

**Plan**

1. Neutral wrist splint to maintain to be worn at bedtime
2. Vitamin $B_6$ 100 mg PO BID
3. Physical therapy

# PHYSICAL THERAPY

The patient is a 34-year-old female who presents with right hand tingling and numbness in her first through third fingers that started 3 months ago. The patient is a right-handed administrative assistant. The patient's symptoms have progressively gotten worse over the past month and she recently went to the physician who referred her to physical therapy.

**Scale:** 0/10 pain

**Increase pain:** sleeping at night; typing on the computer

**Decrease pain:** rest

## Range of Motion

**Wrist**

Wrist flexion: WNL increased tingling and numbness
Wrist extension: 30 degrees
Radial deviation: WNL
Ulna deviation: WNL
Supination: 30 degrees
Pronation: WNL

**Elbow**

Flexion: WNL
Extension: –5 degrees

**Shoulder**

WNL

**Joint play**

WNL

**Special tests**

Phalen's +
Scalene compression test: + (with referral into first to third digit)

**Neurodynamic assessment**

Median nerve

**Tight tender points/soft tissue restrictions**

Right thenar eminence—trigger points
Right subscapularis—trigger points (with referral into first to third digit)
Right pronator teres—myofascial restrictions (with referral into first to third digit)
Right transverse carpal ligament—myofascial restriction

**Ergonomics**

WNL

## ASSESSMENT

The patient presents with right tingling and numbness into the first to third digits that is indicative of carpal tunnel syndrome.

### Plan

Self–myofascial release/corrective flexibility/corrective exercises/corrective manual therapy/modalities

---

### Self–Myofascial Release

**1.** None

---

### Corrective Flexibility

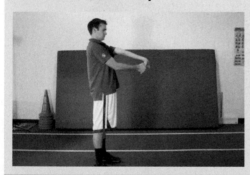

**FIGURE 11.1.** Neurodynamic: median nerve.

---

### Corrective Exercise

**3.** Phase 1: Pain management phase—exercise should be limited secondary to the repetitive trauma of the elbow for the first 2 weeks until pain is resolved.
**4.** Phase 2: Exercise is slowly introduced.

*(continued)*

## Corrective Exercise (*continued*)

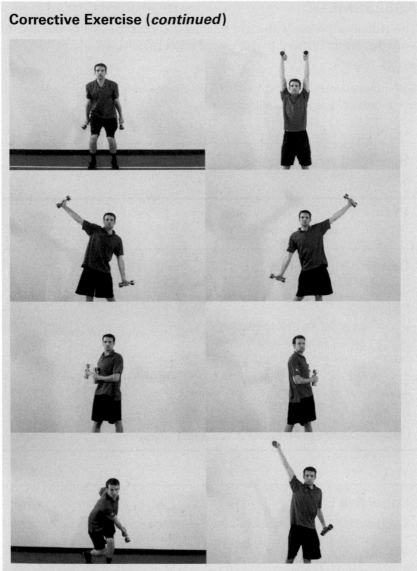

**FIGURE 11.2A.** Shoulder matrix.

(*continued*)

## Corrective Exercise (*continued*)

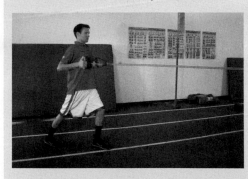

**FIGURE 11.2B.** Pull: split stance/ theraband/two arms.

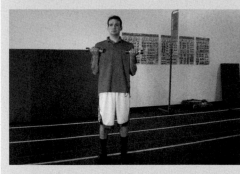

**FIGURE 11.2C.** Bicep curls: palm up.

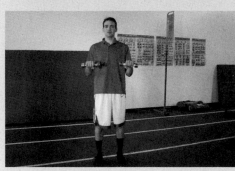

**FIGURE 11.2D.** Bicep curls: palm down.

## Manual Therapy

1. Warming technique: brachioradialis; flexor carpi ulnaris; wrist flexors; medial intermuscular septum; biceps brachii
2. Inhibitory technique: right brachioradialis; flexor carpi ulnaris; biceps brachii
3. Activation technique: right brachioradialis; flexor carpi ulnaris
4. Elongation technique: pronator teres; flexor carpi ulnaris; biceps brachii

## Modalities: prn

1. Ice pack
2. US pulse

## Home Exercise Program

1. Neurodynamic: median nerve
2. Ice pack

Orthopedic and Rehabilitation Associates
Orthopedic Street
Omaha, OH
(555) 555-5555
Fax. (666) 666-7777

PATIENT: *Mr. Lf*
DATE: *2009*

## ORTHOPAEDIC REHABILITATION PRESCRIPTION

| REHAB THERAPIES | ☒ PT | ☐ OT | ☐ SESSIONS/WK _2_ |
| --- | --- | --- | --- |

TOTAL _12_

☒ NEW DIAGNOSIS    ☐ RE-EVALUATION    ☒ OUTPATIENT

DIAGNOSIS1 _Carpal Tunnel Syndrome_
ICD _____

DIAGNOSIS2 _____
ICD _____

PREGNANT? ☐ YES ☒ NO        PERTINENT MEDICAL HISTORY: _None_

GOALS:
MD/DO: ☒ INCREASE MOBILITY ☒ INCREASE ADL ☒ INCREASE STRENGTH ☒ DECREASE PAIN

PRECAUTIONS: ☐ CARDIAC    MAX-SBP ____ DBP ____ HR ____

ABOVE BASELINE    ☐ DIABETES: HYPER/HYPOGLYCEMIA ☐ ORTHOSTASIS
☐ OTHER _____

WEIGHT BEARING: ☐ WBAT ☐ TTWB ☐ NWB
TO: _____

MODALITIES: ☐ ULTRASOUND TO: _R wrist and hand x 1 min_
☐ E-STIM    TO: _R wrist and hand x 1 B/L_

B/L _____

☐ FLUID THERAPY    ☐ JOBST    ☐ PARAFFIN
TO: _____

☐ ICE    TO: _10 min to R elbow_

B/L _____

☐ HOTPACKS    TO: _10 min to R elbow_
☐ EXERCISES ☐ PROM ☐ AAROM ☐ AROM
TO: _B/L UE_
☒ PRE's ☐ ISOMETRICS ☐ ISOKINETICS
TO: _B/L UE_
☐ SLIDEBOARD ☐ PLYOMETRICS ☐ MODIFIED KNEE BEND
☐ STEPUPS
☐ LUMBAR STABILIZATION ☐ WILLIAM's ☐ McKENZIE ☒ CERVICAL EXERCISES
☐ RELAXATION ☐ COORDINATION

MANUAL: ☒ CONTRACT RELAX ☐ CRANIOSACRAL ☒ JONES/C-STRAIN ☒ SOFT
TISSUE MOBILIZATION
☒ STRETCHING ☒ MASSAGE ☒ MYOF AS RELEASE ☒ SPRAY/STRETCH
TO: _UE B/L_

EDUCATION: ☒ MOBILITY: ☐ TRANSFERS ☒ ADL ☒ HEP ☐ ENERGY CONSERV
☐ WORK HARDENING ☒ BIOMECHANICS ☐ 1
HANDED TECHNIQUES
☐ GAIT TRAINING ☐ FINE MOTOR ☐ COORD/BALANCE
OTHER: _____
_____
_____

ADL-ACTIVITIES OF DAILY LIVING    AAROM-ACTIVE/ASSISTIVE RANGE OF MOTION   DBP-
DIASTOLIC BLOOD PRESSURE
SBP-SYSTOLIC BLOOD PRESSURE    HR-HEART RATE    HEP-HOME EXERCISE PROGRAM
NWB-NON-WEIGHT BEARING
PRE's-PROGRESSIVE RESISTIVE EXERCISES    WBAT-WEIGHT BEARING AS TOLERATED
ROM-RANGE OF MOTION

The above is medically necessary to decrease debility and achieve ADL independence. Also to:
☒ decrease pain, ☒ improve strength/endurance, ☒ improve balance coordination, ☐ improve gait,
☐ improve transfers,
Other _____

PHYSICIAN'S SIGNATURE _____ DATE _____

# CASE **12**

## DE QUERVAIN TENOSYNOVITIS

**CC:** Left wrist pain

**HPI:** Ms. L is 28 years old and recently gave birth to a healthy baby boy. Her son is now 6 months old. She is doing well except that her left wrist has been hurting for the last 4 months. The pain is on the lateral aspect of her wrist, over the first dorsal compartment of the wrist. No numbness, tingling, or burning. No weakness. No neck pain or radiating symptoms. She has not done anything about the pain. She wanted to come to the doctor sooner but has been too busy with her son and was hoping the pain would just get better. Instead it has gotten worse. She rates the pain as 1/10 when resting but 5/10 when picking up her son, which she naturally has to do a lot. She is breast-feeding and does not want to take any pain medications. She denies any trauma to the wrist or arm.

**PMHx:** None

**PSHx:** None

**Meds:** None

**Allergies:** NKDA

**Social:** No tobacco. No EtOH

**ROS:** Noncontributory

## PHYSICAL EXAMINATION

On exam, Ms. L is a well-developed female who looks her stated age. BP: 108/64, P: 68, RR: 14. She has 5/5 strength, intact sensation, and 2+ biceps, triceps, and brachioradialis reflexes in her upper extremities bilaterally. She has a positive left Finkelstein test and tenderness over the first dorsal wrist compartment. No swelling is evident. 2+ distal pulses are palpated bilaterally.

## Impression

Right de Quervain tenosynovitis

## Plan

1. Thumb spica splint
2. Physical therapy

# PHYSICAL THERAPY

The patient is a 28-year-old female who presents with left wrist pain that started 4 months ago. The patient's symptoms have progressively gotten worse over the past month and she recently went to the physician who referred her to physical therapy.

**Scale:** 1/10 pain at rest to 5/10

**Increase pain:** when picking up her son; knitting; tying her shoelaces; pouring orange juice in the morning

**Decrease pain:** rest; ice

## Range of Motion

**Wrist**

Wrist flexion: WNL

Wrist extension: WNL

Radial deviation: WNL

Ulna deviation: WNL with pain

Supination: WNL

Pronation: WNL

Opposition: WNL with pain

Elbow: WNL

**Shoulder**

WNL

**Joint play**

WNL

**Special tests**

Finkelstein +

**Manual muscle testing**

4/5 brachioradialis with pain

**Neurodynamic assessment**

WNL

**Tight tender points/soft tissue restrictions**

Left brachioradialis—trigger points

Left extensor pollicis longus and abductor pollicis—myofascial restrictions

**Ergonomics**

WNL

## ASSESSMENT

The patient presents with left wrist pain with a positive Finkelstein's, both signs and sx are indicative of de Quervain tenosynovitis, secondary to pattern overload from picking up her son who is an infant. Trigger points and muscle weakness in the brachioradialis are contributing symptoms.

### Plan

Self–myofascial release/corrective flexibility/corrective exercises/corrective manual therapy/modalities

---

### Self Myofascial Release
1. None

---

### Corrective Flexibility
1. None

---

### Corrective Exercise
1. Phase 1: Pain Management Phase—Exercise should be limited secondary to the repetitive trauma of the elbow for the first 2 weeks until pain is resolved.
2. Phase 2: Exercise is slowly introduced.

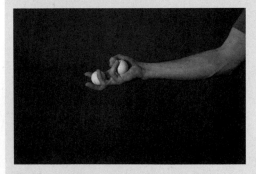

**FIG. 12.1A.** Golf ball rolling.

(*continued*)

## Corrective Exercise (*continued*)

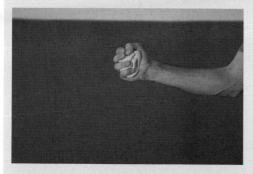

**FIG. 12.1B.** Thera-puddy squeeze.

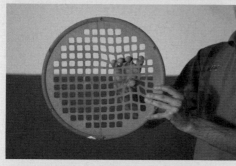

**FIG. 12.1C.** Thera-web squeeze.

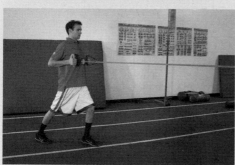

**FIG. 12.1D.** Pull: split stance/ theraband/two arms.

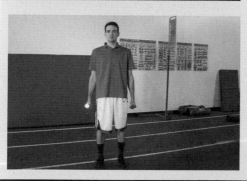

**FIG. 12.1E.** Hammer curls (bicep curl with thumb up).

## Manual Therapy

1. Warming technique: left brachioradialis; wrist extensors; wrist flexors; extensor pollicis longus; abductor pollicis
2. Inhibitory technique: left brachioradialis
3. Activation technique: left brachioradialis
4. Elongation technique: extensor pollicis longus; abductor pollicis

## Modalities: prn

1. Ice pack
2. US pulse

## Home Exercise Program

1. Ice pack: as needed

Orthopedic and Rehabilitation Associates
Orthopedic Street
Omaha, OH
(555) 555-5555
Fax. (666) 666-7777

PATIENT: _Ms. L_
DATE: _2009_

## ORTHOPAEDIC REHABILITATION PRESCRIPTION

REHAB THERAPIES    ☒ PT    ☐ OT    ☐ SESSIONS/WK _2_
TOTAL _12_

☒ NEW DIAGNOSIS    ☐ RE-EVALUATION    ☒ OUTPATIENT

DIAGNOSIS1 _Carpal Tunnel Syndrome_
ICD _____

DIAGNOSIS2 _____
ICD _____

PREGNANT? ☐ YES  ☒ NO          PERTINENTMEDICALHISTORY: _None_

GOALS:
MD/DO: ☒ INCREASE MOBILITY ☒ INCREASE ADL ☒ INCREASE STRENGTH ☒ DECREASE PAIN

PRECAUTIONS: ☐ CARDIAC    MAX-SBP _____ DBP _____ HR _____
ABOVE BASELINE    ☐ DIABETES: HYPER/HYPOGLYCEMIA ☐ ORTHOSTASIS
☐ OTHER _____
WEIGHT BEARING:    ☐ WBAT    ☐ TTWB    ☐ NWB
TO: _____
MODALITIES: ☐ ULTRASOUND TO: _R wrist and hand x 1 min_
          ☐ E-STIM    TO: _R wrist and hand x 1 min B/L_
B/L _____
          ☐ FLUID THERAPY       ☐ JOBST       ☐ PARAFFIN
     TO: _____
          ☐ ICE    TO: _10 min to R elbow_
B/L _____
          ☐ HOTPACKS    TO: _10 min to R elbow_
          ☐ EXERCISES ☐ PROM ☐ AAROM ☐ AROM
     TO: _B/L UE_
          ☒ PRE's    ☐ ISOMETRICS    ☐ ISOKINETICS
     TO: _B/L UE_
          ☐ SLIDEBOARD ☐ PLYOMETRICS ☐ MODIFIED KNEE BEND
☐ STEPUPS
☐ LUMBAR STABILIZATION ☐ WILLIAM's ☐ McKENZIE ☒ CERVICAL EXERCISES
☐ RELAXATION ☐ COORDINATION
MANUAL: ☒ CONTRACT RELAX ☐ CRANIOSACRAL ☒ JONES/C-STRAIN ☒ SOFT
TISSUE MOBILIZATION
          ☒ STRETCHING ☒ MASSAGE ☒ MYOF AS RELEASE ☒ SPRAY/STRETCH
     TO: _UE B/L_
EDUCATION: ☒ MOBILITY: ☐ TRANSFERS ☒ ADL ☒ HEP ☐ ENERGY CONSERV
     ☐ WORK HARDENING ☒ BIOMECHANICS ☐ 1
HANDED TECHNIQUES
☐ GAIT TRAINING ☐ FINE MOTOR ☐ COORD/BALANCE
OTHER: _____
_____
_____

ADL-ACTIVITIES OF DAILY LIVING    AAROM-ACTIVE/ASSISTIVERANGEOFMOTION   DBP-
DIASTOLIC BLOOD PRESSURE
SBP-SYSTOLIC BLOOD PRESSURE   HR-HEART RATE   HEP-HOME EXERCISE PROGRAM
NWB-NON-WEIGHT BEARING
PRE's-PROGRESSIVE RESISTIVE EXERCISES   WBAT-WEIGHT BEARING AS TOLERATED
ROM-RANGE OF MOTION

The above is medically necessary to decrease debility and achieve ADL independence. Also to:
☒ decrease pain, ☒ improve strength/endurance, ☒ improve balance coordination, ☐ improve gait,
☐ improve transfers,
Other _____

PHYSICIAN'S SIGNATURE _____ DATE _____

# PART 5

## THORACIC PAIN

# CASE **13**

## MID BACK MYOFASCIAL PAIN

**CC:** Upper back pain

**HPI:** Ms. L is a 38-year-old office administrator who complains of constant mid back pain for the last 2 years. She says that the pain began gradually and has been getting worse. It is particularly bad at work. It gets somewhat better over the weekend but then starts up again on Monday. She does not believe that it is stress-related, exactly, but sitting still at the desk all day exacerbates the pain. During the weekend, she is outside with her kids and moving around. During the week, the pain is worse when at her desk. She tries to get up and move around while at work but it does not help. No radiation of symptoms into the upper or lower extremities bilaterally. No numbness or tingling. The pain is described as "deep and achy."

**PMHx:** Depression

**PSHx:** Appendectomy

**Meds:** Paxil, Advil prn

**Allergies:** NKDA

**Social:** No tobacco; social EtOH

**ROS:** Noncontributory

## PHYSICAL EXAMINATION

On exam, Ms. L is an overweight female who looks her stated age. BP: 142/90, P: 72, RR: 14  Pain is present with trunk flexion and extension. She has 5/5 strength, intact sensation, and 2+ biceps, triceps, brachioradialis, patella, and Achilles reflexes bilaterally. No pathologic reflexes are elicited. Tenderness is noted along the paraspinals from T4 to T12 bilaterally. No specific trigger points are elicited. No bony tenderness is found. 2+ distal pulses are palpated bilaterally.

## Impression

Myofascial thoracic pain

**Plan**

**1.** Physical therapy

## PHYSICAL THERAPY

The patient is a 38-years-old female who presents with mid back pain that started 2 years ago. The pain has progressively gotten worse over time and currently presenting as a deep ache. Recently, the patient went to the physician who referred the patient to physical therapy.

**Scale:** 6–7/10

**Increase pain:** prolonged sitting >20 minutes; working; driving; forward and backward bending

**Decrease pain:** lying supine

### Range of Motion

**Thoracic spine**

T/S rotation left: 75% limited

T/S rotation right: 75% limited

T/S flexion: WNL

T/S extension: 75% limited

**Shoulder**

Shoulder flexion right: 130 degrees

Shoulder flexion left: 130 degrees

**Joint play**

T/S 2/6

**Special tests**

T/S reversal against wall +

**Manual muscle testing**

4/5 bilateral rhomboids

**Neurodynamic assessment**

WNL

**Tight tender points/soft tissue restrictions**

Bilateral spinalis/iliocostalis/longissimus thoracic; rhomboids—trigger points

Bilateral latissimus dorsi; pectoralis major—myofascial restrictions

**Ergonomics**

Poor

## ASSESSMENT

The patient presents with a deep ache into her thoracic spine. The patient has poor ergonomics and poor posture. There is a decreased T/S reversal secondary decreased joint play in the T/S. Weakness noted in the rhomboids and tight tender points in the spinalis, longissimus, and iliocostalis erectors and myofascial restriction in pectoralis major and latissimus dorsi all contributing to her pain and deep ache.

### Plan

Self–myofascial release/corrective flexibility/corrective exercises/corrective manual therapy/modalities

### Self–Myofascial Release

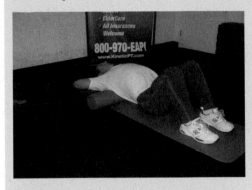

**FIGURE 13.1A.** Foam roll: T/S perpendicular.

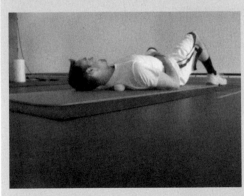

**FIGURE 13.1B.** Tennis ball roll: bilateral rhomboids.

## Corrective Flexibility

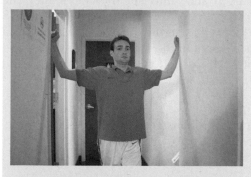

**FIGURE 13.2A.** Static: bilateral pectoralis major in doorway.

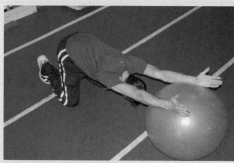

**FIGURE 13.2B.** Static: bilateral latissimus dorsi stretch/ physioball.

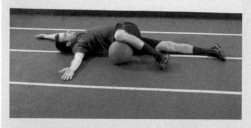

**FIGURE 13.2C.** Active: T/S rotation/ sideline.

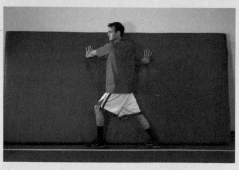

**FIGURE 13.2D.** Active: T/S rotation/ against wall.

## Corrective Exercise

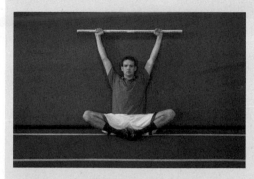

**FIGURE 13.3A.** Wall sit: overhead press.

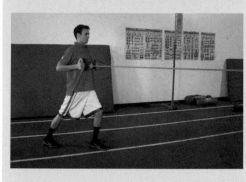

**FIGURE 13.3B.** Pull: SpS/theraband/two arms.

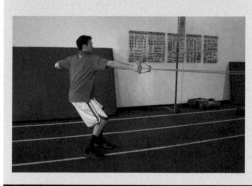

**FIGURE 13.3C.** Pull: PS/theraband/total body rotation.

## Manual Therapy

**1.** Warming technique: thoracic extensors
**2.** Inhibitory technique: thoracic extensors
**3.** Elongation technique: bilateral latissimus dorsi; pectoralis major
**4.** Joint mobilizations: T/S

## Modalities: prn

## Home Exercise Program

**1.** Static: bilateral pectoralis major; latissimus dorsi

Orthopedic and Rehabilitation Associates
Orthopedic Street
Omaha, OH
(555) 555-5555
Fax. (666) 666-7777

PATIENT ___
DATE: 2009

## ORTHOPAEDIC REHABILITATION PRESCRIPTION

| REHAB THERAPIES | ☒ PT | ☐ OT | ☐ SESSIONS/WK _2_ |
| TOTAL _12_ | | | |

☒ NEW DIAGNOSIS    ☐ RE-EVALUATION    ☒ OUTPATIENT

DIAGNOSIS1 _Myofascial thoracic back pain_
    ICD _____

DIAGNOSIS2 _____
    ICD _____

PREGNANT? ☐ YES ☒ NO      PERTINENTMEDICALHISTORY: _None_

GOALS:
MD/DO: ☒ INCREASE MOBILITY ☒ INCREASE ADL ☒ INCREASE STRENGTH ☒ DECREASE PAIN

PRECAUTIONS: ☐ CARDIAC    MAX-SBP _____ DBP _____ HR _____
ABOVE BASELINE    ☐ DIABETES: HYPER/HYPOGLYCEMIA ☐ ORTHOSTASIS
☐ OTHER _____
WEIGHT BEARING:    ☐ WBAT    ☐ TTWB    ☐ NWB
    TO: _____
MODALITIES: ☐ ULTRASOUND TO: _Thoracic paraspinals x 7 min_
              ☐ E-STIM    TO: _Thoracic paraspinals x 7 min B/L_

B/L _____
        ☐ FLUID THERAPY    ☐ JOBST    ☐ PARAFFIN
    TO: _____
        ☐ ICE    TO: _10 min to thoracic paraspinals_
B/L _____
        ☐ HOTPACKS    TO: _10 min to thoracic paraspinals_
        ☐ EXERCISES ☐ PROM ☐ AAROM ☐ AROM
    TO: _B/L LE_
        ☒ PRE's ☐ ISOMETRICS ☐ ISOKINETICS
    TO: _B/L LE_
        ☐ SLIDEBOARD ☐ PLYOMETRICS ☐ MODIFIED KNEE BEND
☐ STEPUPS
☒ LUMBAH STABILIZATION ☐ WILLIAM's ☐ McKENZIE ☒ CERVICAL EXERCISES
☐ RELAXATION ☐ COORDINATION
MANUAL: ☒ CONTRACT RELAX ☐ CRANIOSACRAL ☒ JONES/C-STRAIN ☒ SOFT
TISSUE MOBILIZATION
        ☒ STRETCHING ☒ MASSAGE ☒ MYOF AS RELEASE ☒ SPRAY/STRETCH
    TO: _UE B/L_
EDUCATION: ☒ MOBILITY: ☐ TRANSFERS ☒ ADL ☒ HEP ☐ ENERGY CONSERV
☐ WORK HARDENING ☒ BIOMECHANICS ☐ 1
HANDED TECHNIQUES
☐ GAIT TRAINING ☐ FINE MOTOR ☐ COORD/BALANCE
OTHER: _____
_____
_____

ADL-ACTIVITIES OF DAILY LIVING    AAROM-ACTIVE/ASSISTIVERANGEOFMOTION    DBP-
DIASTOLIC BLOOD PRESSURE
SBP-SYSTOLIC BLOOD PRESSURE    HR-HEART RATE    HEP-HOME EXERCISE PROGRAM
NWB-NON-WEIGHT BEARING
PRE's-PROGRESSIVE RESISTIVE EXERCISES    WBAT-WEIGHT BEARING AS TOLERATED
ROM-RANGE OF MOTION

The above is medically necessary to decrease debility and achieve ADL independence. Also to:
☒ decrease pain, ☒ improve strength/endurance, ☒ improve balance coordination, ☐ improve gait,
☐ improve transfers,
Other _____

PHYSICIAN'S SIGNATURE _____    DATE _____

# CASE 14

# THORACIC COMPRESSION FRACTURE

**CC:** Back pain

**HPI:** Mr. G is 76 years old and complains of severe (7/10) back pain for the last 2 weeks. He does not "like going to doctors" so he tried to give the pain time and rest and see if things would get better. But the pain has persisted and he wants to do something about it. The pain began suddenly when he bent over to open a window. He thought he "threw the back out" as he had in the past, but this time it "felt different." Denies any radiation of symptoms into his lower extremities bilaterally. No numbness, tingling, or burning. No weakness. The pain is "sharp" and "stabbing," and worse with sitting or bending forward. The pain is located at the bottom of his thoracic spine. He hates taking pain medications but has been taking Tylenol, which does not help.

**PMHx:** BPH, HTN, high cholesterol

**PSHx:** Cataract surgery

**Meds:** Flomax, Toprol XL, Lipitor, Tylenol

**Allergies:** NKDA

**Social:** Quit smoking in 1984; social EtOH

**ROS:** Noncontributory

## PHYSICAL EXAMINATION

On exam, Mr. G is in mild discomfort while sitting and appears his stated age. BP: 140/88, P: 76, RR: 14. Pain with trunk flexion. Pain is somewhat reduced with trunk extension. He has 5/5 strength in his lower extremities, bilaterally, though has pain with resisted muscle testing. His sensation in his lower extremities is intact bilaterally. No pathologic reflexes are elicited. Marked tenderness is noted over the T12 spinous process. The paraspinals are mildly tender. 2+ LE distal pulses are palpated bilaterally.

### Impression

Thoracic compression fracture

### Plan

**1.** X-rays
**2.** Physical therapy
**3.** D/C Tylenol. Start Vicodin prn

## PHYSICAL THERAPY

The patient is a 76-year-old male who presents with mid back pain that started 2 weeks ago. The pain started suddenly after bending forward to open the window. The pain is sharp and stabbing in nature.
**Scale:** 7/10
**Increase pain:** prolonged sitting >10 minutes; driving; forward and backward bending
**Decrease pain:** lying sideline

### Range of Motion

**Thoracic spine**
T/S rotation left: 50% limited
T/S rotation right: 50% limited
T/S flexion: WNL
T/S extension: 75% limited
**Shoulder**
Shoulder flexion right: 120 degrees
Shoulder flexion left: 120 degrees
**Joint play**
N/A secondary to spinal fracture
**Special tests**
T/S reversal against wall +
**Manual muscle testing**
4–/5 bilateral rhomboids with pain
**Neurodynamic assessment**
WNL
**Tight tender points/soft tissue restrictions**
Bilateral spinalis/iliocostalis/longissimus thoracic; rhomboids—trigger points
Bilateral latissimus dorsi; pectoralis major—myofascial restrictions

**Ergonomics**
Poor

## ASSESSMENT

The patient presents with a T/S compression fracture. The patient has poor ergonomics and poor posture. There is a decreased T/S reversal secondary to pain and myofascial restrictions in the latissimus dorsi and pectoralis major. Weakness noted in the rhomboids.

### Plan

Self–myofascial release/corrective flexibility/corrective exercises/corrective manual therapy/modalities

---

### Corrective Flexibility

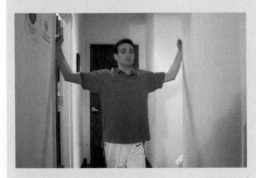

**FIGURE 14.1A.** Static: bilateral pectoralis major in doorway.

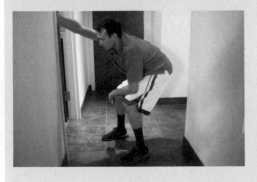

**FIGURE 14.1B.** Static: bilateral latissimus dorsi stretch/doorway.

(*continued*)

## Corrective Flexibility (*continued*)

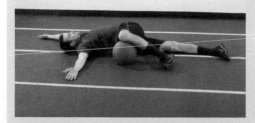

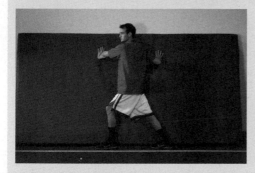

**FIGURE 14.1C.** Active: T/S rotation/sideline.

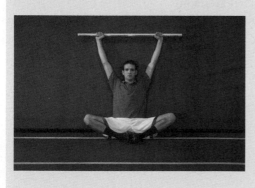

**FIGURE 14.1D.** Active: T/S rotation/against wall.

## Corrective Exercise

**FIGURE 14.2A.** Wall sit: overhead press.

(*continued*)

## Corrective Exercise (*continued*)

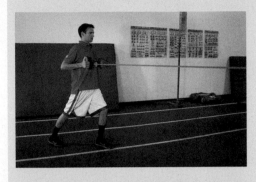

**FIGURE 14.2B.** Pull: SpS/thera-band/two arms.

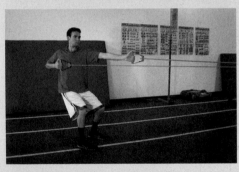

**FIGURE 14.2C.** Pull: PS/thera-band/total body rotation.

### Manual Therapy
1. Warming technique: thoracic extensors
2. Elongation technique: bilateral latissimus dorsi; pectoralis major

### Modalities: prn
1. Moist heat: pretreatment as needed

### Home Exercise Program
1. Static: bilateral pectoralis major; latissimus dorsi

Orthopedic and Rehabilitation Associates
Orthopedic Street
Omaha, OH
(555) 555-5555
Fax. (666) 666-7777

PATIENT: *Mr. G*
DATE: *2009*

## ORTHOPAEDIC REHABILITATION PRESCRIPTION

**REHAB THERAPIES** ☒ PT ☐ OT ☐ SESSIONS/WK *2*
TOTAL *12*

☒ NEW DIAGNOSIS ☐ RE-EVALUATION ☒ OUTPATIENT

DIAGNOSIS1 *Compression fracture*
　ICD _____

DIAGNOSIS2 _____
　ICD _____

PREGNANT? ☐ YES ☒ NO 　　PERTINENTMEDICALHISTORY: *HTN*

GOALS:
MD/DO: ☒ INCREASE MOBILITY ☒ INCREASE ADL ☒ INCREASE STRENGTH ☒ DECREASE PAIN

PRECAUTIONS: ☐ CARDIAC 　MAX-SBP *20* DBP *10* HR *20*
ABOVE BASELINE 　☐ DIABETES: HYPER/HYPOGLYCEMIA ☐ ORTHOSTASIS
☐ OTHER _____
WEIGHT BEARING: ☐ WBAT ☐ TTWB ☐ NWB
　TO: _____
MODALITIES: ☐ ULTRASOUND TO: *Thoracic paraspinals x 1 min*
　　　☐ E-STIM 　TO: *Thoracic paraspinals x 1 min B/L*
B/L _____
　☐ FLUID THERAPY 　☐ JOBST 　☐ PARAFFIN
　TO: _____
　☐ ICE 　TO: *10 min to thoracic paraspinals*
B/L _____
　☐ HOTPACKS 　TO: *10 min to thoracic paraspinals*
　☐ EXERCISES ☐ PROM ☐ AAROM ☐ AROM
　TO: *B/L LE*
　☒ PRE's ☐ ISOMETRICS ☐ ISOKINETICS
　TO: *B/L LE*
　☐ SLIDEBOARD ☐ PLYOMETRICS ☐ MODIFIED KNEE BEND
☐ STEPUPS
☒ LUMBAR STABILIZATION ☐ WILLIAM's ☒ McKENZIE ☐ CERVICAL EXERCISES
☐ RELAXATION ☐ COORDINATION
MANUAL: ☒ CONTRACT RELAX ☐ CRANIOSACRAL ☒ JONES/C-STRAIN ☒ SOFT
TISSUE MOBILIZATION
　　☒ STRETCHING ☐ MASSAGE ☒ MYOF AS RELEASE ☒ SPRAY/STRETCH
　TO: *UE B/L*
EDUCATION: ☒ MOBILITY: ☐ TRANSFERS ☒ ADL ☒ HEP ☐ ENERGY CONSERV
　☐ WORK HARDENING ☒ BIOMECHANICS ☐ 1
HANDED TECHNIQUES
　☐ GAIT TRAINING ☐ FINE MOTOR ☐ COORD/BALANCE
OTHER: _____
_____
_____

ADL-ACTIVITIES OF DAILY LIVING 　AAROM-ACTIVE/ASSISTIVERANGEOFMOTION 　DBP-
DIASTOLIC BLOOD PRESSURE
SBP-SYSTOLIC BLOOD PRESSURE 　HR-HEART RATE 　HEP-HOME EXERCISE PROGRAM
NWB-NON-WEIGHT BEARING
PRE's-PROGRESSIVE RESISTIVE EXERCISES 　WBAT-WEIGHT BEARING AS TOLERATED
ROM-RANGE OF MOTION

The above is medically necessary to decrease debility and achieve ADL independence. Also to:
☒ decrease pain, ☒ improve strength/endurance, ☒ improve balance coordination, ☒ improve gait,
☐ improve transfers,
Other _____

PHYSICIAN'S SIGNATURE _____ DATE _____

# PART 6

## LUMBOSACRAL SPINE

# CASE 15

## LUMBAR STRAIN

**CC:** Lower back pain

**HPI:** Mr. Z is a 38-year-old investment banker who presents on Monday having hurt his left lower back after playing basketball on Saturday. He does not remember a particular injury during his game, but that night his back was achy. He woke up Sunday in "excruciating pain." Today, the pain is only modestly improved. No radiation of symptoms. No numbness, tingling, burning, or weakness. No change in bowel or bladder. The pain is somewhat worse with sitting but is painful all the time. The pain stretches across his entire back, but in the left side is much worse. He rates the pain 7/10. He has been taking Advil and extra strength Tylenol "around the clock" with minimal relief. He wants to ease the pain but does not want to take a narcotic because he needs "to stay alert."

**PMHx:** None

**PSHx:** None

**Meds:** Advil, Tylenol prn

**Allergies:** NKDA

**Social:** No smoking; social EtOH

**ROS:** Noncontributory

## PHYSICAL EXAMINATION

On exam, Mr. Z is in moderate discomfort. BP: 144/86, P: 80, RR: 14. He has increased pain with trunk flexion and overall limited trunk mobility secondary to pain. He has 5/5 strength in his lower extremities,

**111**

bilaterally, though has pain with resisted muscle testing. His sensation in his lower extremities is intact bilaterally. 2+ reflexes in the patella and Achilles are elicited bilaterally. No pathologic reflexes are elicited. He has discomfort while switching positions. Tenderness is noted over the bilateral lumbar paraspinals, L > R. 2+ distal pulses are palpated bilaterally.

## Impression

Acute lumbar strain

## Plan

1. Physical therapy
2. D/C Advil and Tylenol. Instead, Voltaren 75 mg PO BID and Ultracet 1 PO TID prn

# PHYSICAL THERAPY

The patient is a 38-year-old male who presents with left lower back pain that started several days ago after playing basketball. The day after playing basketball the patient woke up with severe low back pain. The patient feels increased pain with sit-to-stand and feels hunched over.
**Scale:** 7/10
**Increase pain:** sitting; constant in nature; sitting to standing
**Decrease pain:** Advil and extra strength Tylenol

## Range of Motion

**Lumbar spine**
Flexion: 50% with pain
Extension: 75% with pain
Left sidebending: 75% with pain
Right sidebending: 75% with pain
Left rotation: WNL
Right rotation: WNL
**Thoracic spine**
T/S rotation left: WNL
T/S rotation right: WNL
T/S flexion: WNL
T/S extension: WNL
**Hip**
Left hip extension: –10 degrees
Right hip extension: 0 degree
Bilateral hip internal rotation: 0 degree
**Joint play**
Empty end feel
**Special tests**
Spurling's –

Sideglide –
SLR –
**Manual muscle testing**
Core: 4/5 throughout
Psoas: 4–/5 bilateral with pain
Piriformis: 4–/5 bilateral with pain
**Neurodynamic assessment**
WNL
**Tight tender points/soft tissue restrictions**
Bilateral psoas; iliacus; quadratus lumborum; piriformis—trigger points
Bilateral psoas left > right—myofascial restrictions
**Ergonomics**
Fair secondary to pain

## ASSESSMENT

The patient presents with an acute lumbar spine sprain/strain with trigger points in bilateral psoas; iliacus; quadratus lumborum; and the piriformis. Myofascial restrictions noted in the psoas left > right causing decreased hip extension on the left and the inability to transition from a sitting position to a standing position without increased symptoms and being hunched. Core weakness was noted.

### Plan

Self–myofascial release/corrective flexibility/corrective exercises/corrective manual therapy/modalities

### Self–Myofascial Release

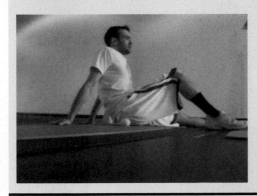

**FIGURE 15.1.** Tennis ball: bilateral piriformis.

## Corrective Flexibility

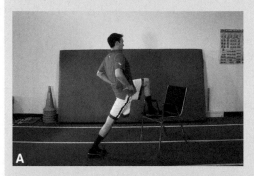

**FIGURE 15.2(A–C).** Static: hip flexor stretch/3D 2:1 ratio left to right.

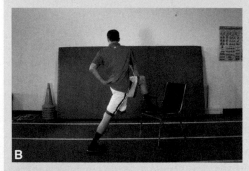

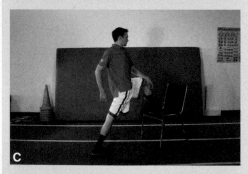

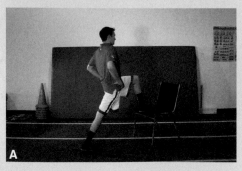

**FIGURE 15.3(A–C).** Active: hip flexor stretch/3D 2:1 ratio left to right.

(*continued*)

## Corrective Flexibility (*continued*)

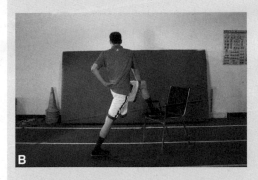

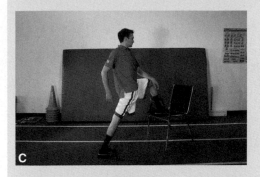

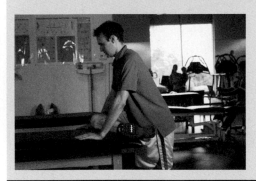

**FIGURE 15.4.** Static: piriformis on bench.

## Corrective Exercise

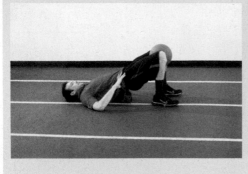

**FIGURE 15.5A.** Bridging: two legs.

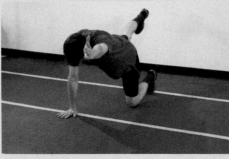

**FIGURE 15.5B.** Quadruped: alternate limb extensions.

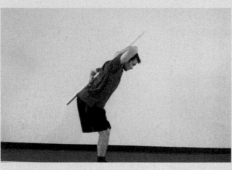

**FIGURE 15.5C.** Deadlift: technique/hip hinge.

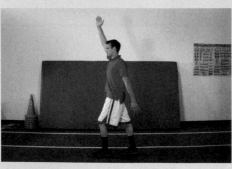

**FIGURE 15.6.** Walk matrix.

(*continued*)

# Corrective Exercise (*continued*)

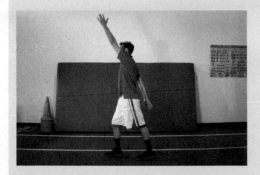

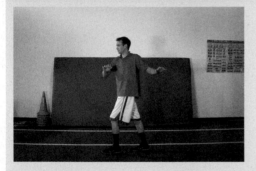

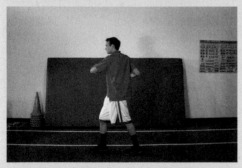

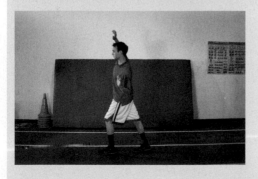

(*continued*)

## Corrective Exercise (*continued*)

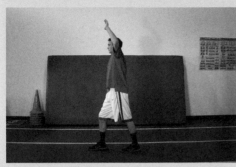

## Manual Therapy

1. Warming technique: lumbar erectors; bilateral piriformis
2. Inhibitory technique: bilateral psoas; quadratus lumborum
3. Elongation technique: left psoas/iliacus

## Modalities: prn

1. Ice as needed

## Home Exercise Program

1. Tennis ball: bilateral piriformis
2. Static: bilateral psoas; piriformis

Orthopedic and Rehabilitation Associates
Orthopedic Street
Omaha, OH
(555) 555-5555
Fax (555) 555-7777

PATIENT: _Mr Z_
DATE: _2009_

## ORTHOPAEDIC REHABILITATION PRESCRIPTION

| _REHAB THERAPIES_ | ☒ PT | ☐ OT | ☐ SESSIONS/WK _2_ |
| --- | --- | --- | --- |

TOTAL _12_

☒ NEW DIAGNOSIS    ☐ RE-EVALUATION    ☒ OUTPATIENT

DIAGNOSIS1 _Compression Fracture_
    ICD _____

DIAGNOSIS2 _____
    ICD _____

PREGNANT? ☐ YES  ☒ NO    PERTINENTMEDICALHISTORY: _None_

GOALS:
MD/DO: ☒ INCREASE MOBILITY  ☒ INCREASE ADL  ☒ INCREASE STRENGTH  ☒ DECREASE PAIN

PRECAUTIONS: ☐ CARDIAC    MAX-SBP _____ DBP _____ HR _____
ABOVE BASELINE    ☐ DIABETES: HYPER/HYPOGLYCEMIA  ☐ ORTHOSTASIS
☐ OTHER _____

WEIGHT BEARING:    ☐ WBAT    ☐ TTWB    ☐ NWB
    TO: _____

MODALITIES: ☐ ULTRASOUND TO: _Lumbar paraspinals x 1 min_
            ☐ E-STIM    TO: _Lumbar paraspinals x 1 min B/L_
B/L _____
            ☐ FLUID THERAPY    ☐ JOBST    ☐ PARAFFIN
    TO: _____
            ☐ ICE    TO: _10 min to lumbar paraspinals_
B/L _____
            ☐ HOTPACKS    TO: _10 min to lumbar paraspinals_
            ☐ EXERCISES  ☐ PROM  ☐ AAROM  ☐ AROM
    TO: _B/L LE_
            ☒ PRE's  ☐ ISOMETRICS  ☐ ISOKINETICS
    TO: _B/L LE_
            ☐ SLIDEBOARD  ☐ PLYOMETRICS  ☐ MODIFIED KNEE BEND
☐ STEPUPS
☒ LUMBAR STABILIZATION  ☐ WILLIAM's  ☒ McKENZIE  ☐ CERVICAL EXERCISES
☐ RELAXATION  ☐ COORDINATION
MANUAL: ☒ CONTRACT RELAX  ☐ CRANIOSACRAL  ☒ JONES/C-STRAIN  ☒ SOFT
TISSUE MOBILIZATION
            ☒ STRETCHING  ☒ MASSAGE  ☒ MYOF AS RELEASE  ☒ SPRAY/STRETCH
    TO: _LE B/L_
EDUCATION: ☒ MOBILITY:  ☐ TRANSFERS  ☒ ADL  ☒ HEP  ☐ ENERGY CONSERV
☐ WORK HARDENING  ☒ BIOMECHANICS  ☐ 1
HANDED TECHNIQUES
☐ GAIT TRAINING  ☐ FINE MOTOR  ☐ COORD/BALANCE
OTHER: _____
_____
_____

ADL-ACTIVITIES OF DAILY LIVING    AAROM-ACTIVE/ASSISTIVERANGEOFMOTION   DBP-
DIASTOLIC BLOOD PRESSURE
SBP-SYSTOLIC BLOOD PRESSURE    HR-HEART RATE    HEP-HOME EXERCISE PROGRAM
NWB-NON-WEIGHT BEARING
PRE's-PROGRESSIVE RESISTIVE EXERCISES    WBAT-WEIGHT BEARING AS TOLERATED
ROM-RANGE OF MOTION

The above is medically necessary to decrease debility and achieve ADL independence. Also to:
☒ decrease pain,  ☒ improve strength/endurance,  ☒ improve balance coordination,  ☒ improve gait,
☐ improve transfers,
Other _____

PHYSICIAN'S SIGNATURE _____ DATE _____

# CASE 16

## SUBACUTE DISCOGENIC LOWER BACK PAIN

**CC:** Back pain

**HPI:** Ms. M is 33 years old and has had lower back pain for 6 weeks. She does not remember a specific inciting event. The pain is "dull" and "aching" and located in the lower back. No radiation of symptoms into the lower extremities bilaterally. No numbness, burning, tingling, or weakness. Pain is worse while sitting, and long car rides are particularly difficult for her. The pain is worse in the morning. Standing and walking make the pain better. No change in bowel or bladder. This is the first time she is coming to a doctor for her symptoms in part because she is trying to start a family and does not want any x-rays. She has not taken any pain medications for the symptoms. She rates the pain as 4/10 on average, and 6/10 after sitting for 10 minutes.

**PMHx:** None
**PSHx:** None
**Meds:** None
**Allergies:** NKDA
**Social:** No smoking; no EtOH
**ROS:** Noncontributory

# PHYSICAL EXAMINATION

On exam, Ms. M is in no acute distress and appears her stated age. BP: 122/76, P: 64, RR: 14. She has increased pain with trunk flexion and no pain with trunk extension. She has 5/5 strength, 2+ patella and Achilles reflexes, and intact sensation in her bilateral lower extremities. No pathologic reflexes are elicited. She has a negative FABER, SLR, and slump test. Tenderness is noted over the bilateral L3-5 paraspinals. The SI joint is not tender. She has pain with maximal simultaneous passive hip and knee flexion. 2+ distal pulses are palpated bilaterally.

## Impression

Subacute discogenic pain

## Plan

1. Physical therapy

# PHYSICAL THERAPY

The patient is a 33-year-old female who presents with lower back pain that started 6 weeks ago with an insidious onset. The pain is dull and achy. The patient went to the physician who referred the patient to physical therapy.

**Scale:** 4/10 on average up to 6/10

**Increase pain:** sitting >10 minutes; mornings; rolling over in bed

**Decrease pain:** walking and moving around

## Range of Motion

**Lumbar spine**

Flexion: 75% with pain

Extension: 75% with pain

Left sidebending: WNL

Right sidebending: WNL

Left rotation: WNL

Right rotation: WNL

**Thoracic spine**

T/S rotation left: WNL

T/S rotation right: WNL

T/S flexion: WNL

T/S extension: WNL

**Hip**

Left hip extension: 0 degree

Right hip extension: 0 degree

Bilateral hip internal rotation: 0 degree

**Joint play**

4/6

**Special tests**
Spurling's –
Sideglide –
SLR –
**Manual muscle testing**
Core: 4/5 throughout
Psoas: 4–/5 bilateral with pain
Piriformis: 4–/5 bilateral with pain
**Neurodynamic assessment**
WNL
**Tight tender points/soft tissue restrictions**
Bilateral psoas; iliacus; quadratus lumborum; piriformis—trigger points
Bilateral psoas left > right—myofascial restrictions
**Ergonomics**
Fair secondary to pain

## ASSESSMENT

The patient presents with an acute lumbar spine sprain/strain with trigger points in bilateral psoas; iliacus; quadratus lumborum; and the piriformis. Myofascial restrictions noted in the psoas left more than right, causing decreased hip extension on the left and the inability to transition from a sitting position to a standing position without increased symptoms and being hunched. Core weakness was noted.

### Plan

Self–myofascial release/corrective flexibility/corrective exercises/ corrective manual therapy/modalities

### Self Myofascial Release

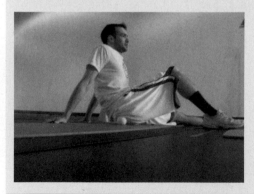

**FIGURE 16.1.** Tennis ball roll: bilateral piriformis.

## Corrective Flexibility

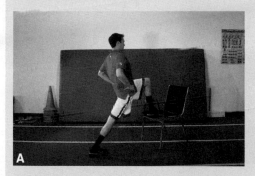

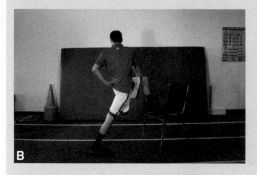

**FIGURE 16.2(A–C).** Static: hip flexor stretch/3D 2:1 ratio left to right.

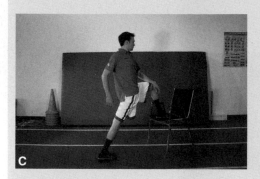

(continued)

## Corrective Flexibility (*continued*)

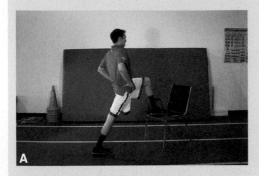

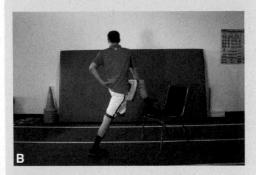

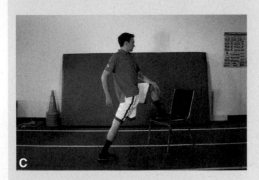

**FIGURE 16.3(A–C).** Active: hip flexor stretch/3D 2:1 ratio left to right.

(*continued*)

## Corrective Flexibility (*continued*)

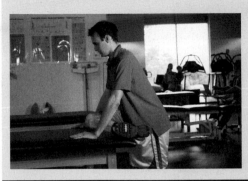

**FIGURE 16.4.** Static: piriformis on bench.

## Corrective Exercise

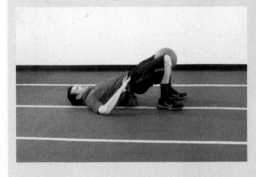

**FIGURE 16.5A.** Bridging two legs.

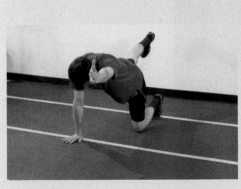

**FIGURE 16.5B.** Quadruped: alternate limb extensions.

(*continued*)

## Corrective Exercise (*continued*)

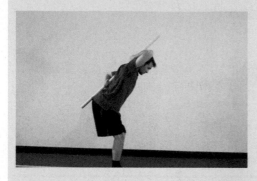

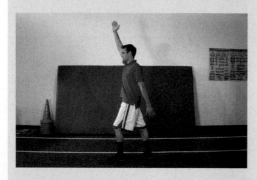

**FIGURE 16.5C.** Deadlift: technique/hip hinge.

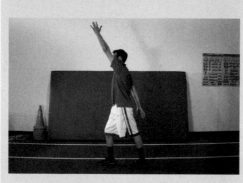

**FIGURE 16.6.** Walk matrix.

*(continued)*

## Corrective Exercise (*continued*)

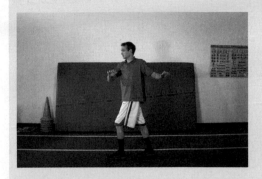

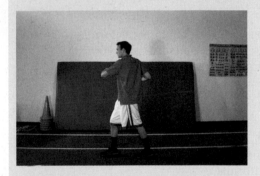

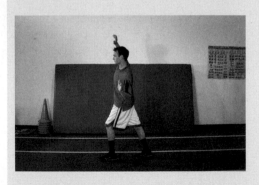

(*continued*)

## Corrective Exercise (*continued*)

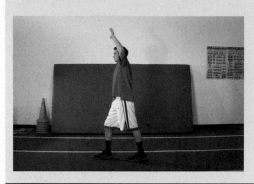

## Manual Therapy

1. Warming technique: lumbar erectors; bilateral piriformis
2. Inhibitory technique: bilateral psoas; quadratus lumborum
3. Elongation technique: left psoas/iliacus

## Modalities: prn

1. Ice as needed

## Home Exercise Program

1. Tennis ball: bilateral piriformis
2. Static: bilateral psoas; piriformis

Orthopedic and Rehabilitation Associates
Orthopedic Street
Omaha, OH
(555) 555-5555
Fax. (666) 666-7777

PATIENT: _Ms. M_
DATE: _2009_

## ORTHOPAEDIC REHABILITATION PRESCRIPTION

| *REHAB THERAPIES* | ☒ PT | ☐ OT | ☐ SESSIONS/WK _2_ |
| --- | --- | --- | --- |

TOTAL _12_

☒ NEW DIAGNOSIS    ☐ RE-EVALUATION    ☒ OUTPATIENT

DIAGNOSIS1 _Subacute discogenic pain_
    ICD _____

DIAGNOSIS2 _____
    ICD _____

PREGNANT? ☐ YES ☒ NO        PERTINENTMEDICALHISTORY: _None_

GOALS:
MD/DO: ☒ INCREASE MOBILITY ☒ INCREASE ADL ☒ INCREASE STRENGTH ☒ DECREASE PAIN

PRECAUTIONS: ☐ CARDIAC    MAX-SBP ____ DBP ____ HR ____

ABOVE BASELINE    ☐ DIABETES: HYPER/HYPOGLYCEMIA ☐ ORTHOSTASIS
☐ OTHER _____

WEIGHT BEARING: ☐ WBAT    ☐ TTWB    ☐ NWB
    TO: _____

MODALITIES: ☐ ULTRASOUND TO: _Lumbar paraspinals x 1 min_
        ☐ E-STIM    TO: _Lumbar paraspinals x 1 min B/L_

B/L _____

    ☐ FLUID THERAPY    ☐ JOBST    ☐ PARAFFIN
    TO: _____
    ☐ ICE    TO: _10 min to lumbar paraspinals_

B/L _____

    ☐ HOTPACKS    TO: _10 min to lumbar paraspinals_
    ☐ EXERCISES ☐ PROM ☐ AAROM ☐ AROM
    TO: _B/L LE_

    ☒ PRE's ☐ ISOMETRICS ☐ ISOKINETICS
    TO: _B/L LE_

    ☐ SLIDEBOARD ☐ PLYOMETRICS ☐ MODIFIED KNEE BEND
☐ STEPUPS
☒ LUMBAR STABILIZATION ☐ WILLIAM's ☒ McKENZIE ☐ CERVICAL EXERCISES
☐ RELAXATION ☐ COORDINATION

MANUAL: ☒ CONTRACT RELAX ☐ CRANIOSACRAL ☒ JONES/C-STRAIN ☒ SOFT
TISSUE MOBILIZATION
        ☒ STRETCHING ☒ MASSAGE ☒ MYOF AS RELEASE ☒ SPRAY/STRETCH
    TO: _LE B/L_

EDUCATION: ☒ MOBILITY: ☐ TRANSFERS ☒ ADL ☐ HEP ☐ ENERGY CONSERV
    ☐ WORK HARDENING ☒ BIOMECHANICS ☐ 1

HANDED TECHNIQUES
    ☐ GAIT TRAINING ☐ FINE MOTOR ☐ COORD/BALANCE
OTHER: _____
_____
_____

ADL-ACTIVITIES OF DAILY LIVING    AAROM-ACTIVE/ASSISTIVERANGEOFMOTION    DBP-
DIASTOLIC BLOOD PRESSURE
SBP-SYSTOLIC BLOOD PRESSURE    HR-HEART RATE    HEP-HOME EXERCISE PROGRAM
NWB-NON-WEIGHT BEARING
PRE's-PROGRESSIVE RESISTIVE EXERCISES    WBAT-WEIGHT BEARING AS TOLERATED
ROM-RANGE OF MOTION

The above is medically necessary to decrease debility and achieve ADL independence. Also to:
☒ decrease pain, ☒ improve strength/endurance, ☒ improve balance coordination, ☒ improve gait,
☐ improve transfers,
Other _____

PHYSICIAN'S SIGNATURE _____    DATE _____

# CASE 17

# CHRONIC DISCOGENIC LOWER BACK PAIN

**CC:** Back pain

**HPI:** Ms. K is 36 years old and has had lower back pain for 4 months. She does not remember a specific inciting event. The pain is "dull" and "aching" and located in the lower back. The pain sometimes radiates to the bilateral buttocks. No numbness, burning, tingling, or weakness. Pain is worse while sitting, and long car rides are particularly difficult. The pain is worse in the morning. She went to her PMD 1 month ago who took x-rays that were "normal" per the patient. She was given a prescription for physical therapy but never went because she decided she should see a spine specialist first. Her PMD also prescribed a muscle relaxant, Flexeril 10 mg PO bedtime, which helps her sleep. During the day she has been taking Tylenol, and this helps take the edge off the pain. No change in bowel or bladder.

**PMHx:** None
**PSHx:** None
**Meds:** OCPs, Flexeril, Tylenol prn
**Allergies:** NKDA
**Social:** No smoking; social EtOH
**ROS:** Noncontributory

## PHYSICAL EXAMINATION

On exam, Ms. K is in no acute distress and appears her stated age. BP: 118/64, P: 60, RR: 14. She has increased pain with trunk flexion and no pain with trunk extension. She has 5/5 strength, 2+ patella and Achilles reflexes, and intact sensation in her bilateral lower extremities. No pathologic reflexes are elicited. She has a negative FABER test. SLR and slump test reproduce back pain bilaterally. Tenderness is noted over the bilateral L4-5 paraspinals. The SI joint is not tender. She has pain with maximal simultaneous passive hip and knee flexion. 2+ distal pulses are palpated bilaterally.

### Impression

Chronic discogenic pain

### Plan

1. MRI
2. Physical therapy

## PHYSICAL THERAPY

The patient is a 36-year-old female who presents with lower back pain that started 4 months ago with an insidious onset. The pain is dull and achy and refers at times into bilateral buttock. The patient went to the physician who took x-rays that showed negative results and was referred to physical therapy.

**Scale:** 7/10

**Increase pain:** sitting >20 minutes; mornings

**Decrease pain:** walking and moving around

### Range of Motion

**Lumbar spine**

Flexion: 50% with pain

Extension: 100% decreases pain

Left sidebending: WNL

Right sidebending: WNL

Left rotation: WNL

Right rotation: WNL

**Thoracic spine**

T/S rotation left: WNL

T/S rotation right: WNL

T/S flexion: WNL

T/S extension: WNL

**Hip**

Left hip extension: WNL

Right hip extension: WNL

Bilateral prone hip internal rotation: –5 degrees

**Joint play**
Bilateral hip posterior capsule 2/6
**Special tests**
Spurling's –
SLR + bilateral
Vasalva –
**Manual muscle testing**
Core: 4/5 throughout
Psoas: 4–/5 bilateral with pain
Piriformis: 4–/5 bilateral with pain
**Neurodynamic assessment**
+ neural tension bilateral on common peroneal nerve
**Tight tender points/soft tissue restrictions**
Bilateral psoas; iliacus; quadratus lumborum; piriformis—trigger points
Bilateral psoas; piriformis—myofascial restrictions
**Ergonomics**
Poor

# ASSESSMENT

The patient presents with chronic discogenic pain with trigger points in bilateral psoas; iliacus; quadratus lumborum; and the piriformis. Myofascial restrictions noted in bilateral psoas and piriformis, which is causing decreased hip internal rotation and is increasing shear force in the lumbar spine secondary to compensatory movement patterns. Spinal extension decreases symptoms. Core weakness was noted.

## Plan

Self–myofascial release/corrective flexibility/corrective exercises/corrective manual therapy/modalities

### Self-Myofascial Release

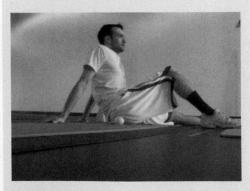

**FIGURE 17.1A.** Tennis ball: bilateral piriformis.

## Corrective Flexibility

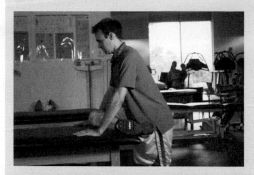

**FIGURE 17.1B.** Static: bilateral piriformis on bench.

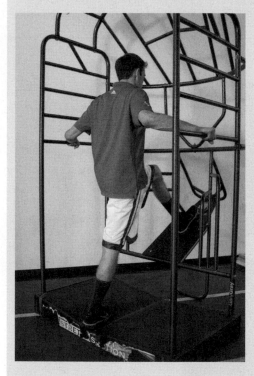

**FIGURE 17.1C.** Active: bilateral psoas.

(*continued*)

## Corrective Flexibility (*continued*)

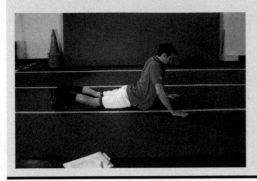

**FIGURE 17.1D.** Active: prone press-up.

## Corrective Exercise

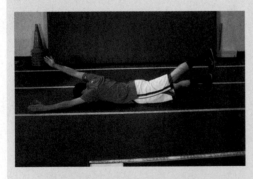

**FIGURE 17.2A.** Prone alternate limb extensions.

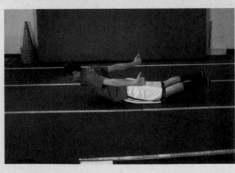

**FIGURE 17.2B.** Prone cobras.

(*continued*)

## Corrective Exercise (*continued*)

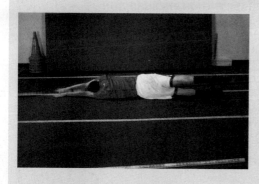

**FIGURE 17.2C.** Rolling: prone to supine with lower extremity drive.

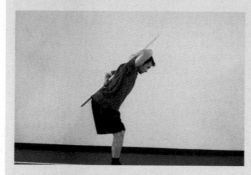

**FIGURE 17.2D.** Deadlift: dowel technique.

### Manual Therapy

1. Warming technique: lumbar erectors; bilateral piriformis
2. Inhibitory technique: bilateral psoas; quadratus lumborum
3. Elongation technique: bilateral piriformis
4. Joint mobilizations: PA mobs L/S0 while doing press-up
5. Joint mobilizations: bilateral hip internal rotation
6. Neuromobilization technique to common peroneal nerve

### Modalities: prn

### Home Exercise Program

1. Tennis ball: bilateral piriformis
2. Static: piriformis
3. Active: prone press-ups

PATIENT: _Ms. K_

DATE: _2009_

## ORTHOPAEDIC REHABILITATION PRESCRIPTION

REHAB THERAPIES   ☒ PT   ☐ OT   ☐ SESSIONS/WK _2_
TOTAL _12_

☐ NEW DIAGNOSIS   ☒ RE-EVALUATION   ☒ OUTPATIENT

DIAGNOSIS1 _Spondylolisthesis_
  ICD _____

DIAGNOSIS2 _Back pain_
  ICD _____

PREGNANT? ☐ YES ☒ NO        PERTINENT MEDICAL HISTORY: _None_

GOALS:
MD/DO: ☒ INCREASE MOBILITY ☒ INCREASE ADL ☒ INCREASE STRENGTH ☒ DECREASE PAIN

PRECAUTIONS: ☐ CARDIAC   MAX-SBP _____ DBP _____ HR _____
ABOVE BASELINE   ☐ DIABETES: HYPER/HYPOGLYCEMIA  ☐ ORTHOSTASIS
☐ OTHER _____
WEIGHT BEARING:   ☐ WBAT   ☐ TTWB   ☐ NWB
  TO: _____

MODALITIES: ☐ ULTRASOUND TO: _Lumbar paraspinals X 1 min_
          ☐ E-STIM   TO: _Lumbar paraspinals X 1 min B/L_
B/L _____
  ☐ FLUID THERAPY   ☐ JOBST   ☐ PARAFFIN
  TO: _____
  ☐ ICE   TO: _____
B/L _____
  ☐ HOTPACKS   TO: _____
  ☐ EXERCISES ☐ PROM ☐ AAROM ☐ AROM
  TO: _B/L LE_
  ☒ PRE's ☐ ISOMETRICS ☐ ISOKINETICS
  TO: _B/L LE_
  ☐ SLIDEBOARD ☐ PLYOMETRICS ☐ MODIFIED KNEE BEND
☐ STEPUPS
☒ LUMBAR STABILIZATION ☒ WILLIAM's ☐ McKENZIE ☐ CERVICAL EXERCISES
☐ RELAXATION ☐ COORDINATION
MANUAL: ☒ CONTRACT RELAX ☐ CRANIOSACRAL ☒ JONES/C-STRAIN ☒ SOFT
TISSUE MOBILIZATION
      ☒ STRETCHING ☒ MASSAGE ☒ MYOFAS RELEASE ☒ SPRAY/STRETCH
  TO: _LE B/L_
EDUCATION: ☒ MOBILITY: ☐ TRANSFERS ☒ ADL ☒ HEP ☐ ENERGY CONSERV
  ☐ WORK HARDENING ☒ BIOMECHANICS ☐ 1 HANDED TECHNIQUES
  ☐ GAIT TRAINING ☐ FINE MOTOR ☐ COORD/BALANCE
OTHER: _____
_____

The above is medically necessary to decrease debility and achieve ADL independence. Also to:
☒ decrease pain, ☒ improve strength/endurance, ☒ improve balance coordination, ☒ improve gait,
☒ improve transfers,
Other _____
PHYSICIAN'S SIGNATURE _____ DATE _____

# CASE 18

# SPONDYLOLISTHESIS

**CC:** Back pain

**HPI:** Ms. A is 43 years old and has had 4 months of axial lower back pain. She does not remember any specific inciting event, though she does mention that she used to be a gymnast and often had back pain toward the end of her college training days. After stopping training, the pain went away and only returned gradually 4 months ago. She is not sure if it is the same character as the old back pain. The pain occasionally radiates into the bilateral buttocks. There is more pain with walking and standing and less pain with sitting. The pain is 5/10 if she goes for a long walk, and it is 2/10 when sitting and talking in the office. Ms. A denies any numbness, burning, tingling, or weakness. She does not take any pain medications and has not had any radiographs of her spine.

**PMHx:** None

**PSHx:** None

**Meds:** None

**Allergies:** NKDA

**Social:** No smoking. No EtOH

**ROS:** Noncontributory

## PHYSICAL EXAMINATION

On exam, Ms. A is pleasant and in no acute distress. BP: 120/82, P: 64, RR: 12. She has increased pain with trunk extension and no pain with trunk flexion. She has 5/5 strength, 2+ patella and Achilles reflexes, and intact sensation in her bilateral lower extremities. No pathologic reflexes are elicited. She has a negative FABER, slump, and SLR test bilaterally. Tenderness is noted over the bilateral L4-5 paraspinals. There is no bony tenderness elicited. The SI joint is not tender. She has no pain with maximal simultaneous passive hip and knee flexion.

Radiographs: X-rays were obtained in the office. Bilateral L5 pars interarticularis fractures and an L5-S1 grade I spondylolisthesis are noted. There is no instability on flexion/extension views. 2 + distal pulses are palpated bilaterally.

## Impression

Grade I spondylolisthesis

**Plan**

1. Physical therapy

# PHYSICAL THERAPY

The patient is a 43-year-old female who presents with lower back pain that started 4 months ago with an insidious onset. The patient was a gymnast in college where she had lower back pain that went away after she stopped training but recently returned. The pain intermittently refers into bilateral buttocks. The patient went to the physician and was referred to physical therapy.

**Scale:** 5/10 at most 2/10 at least

**Increase pain:** 5/10 with standing; walking; spine extension

2/10 with prolonged sitting

**Decrease pain:** lying side line

## Range of Motion

**Lumbar spine**

Flexion: 75% with pain

Extension: 75% with severe pain

Left sidebending: WNL

Right sidebending: WNL

Left rotation: WNL

Right rotation: WNL

**Thoracic spine**

T/S rotation left: WNL

T/S rotation right: WNL

T/S flexion: WNL

T/S extension: WNL

**Hip**

Left hip extension: −10 degrees

Right hip extension: −15 degrees

Bilateral prone hip internal rotation: 0 degree

**Joint play**

WNL

**Special tests**
Spurling's + with pain
SLR –
Vasalva –
**Manual muscle testing**
Core: 4/5 throughout
Psoas: 4/5 bilateral with pain
**Tight tender points/soft tissue restrictions**
Bilateral psoas; iliacus; quadratus lumborum; piriformis—trigger points
Bilateral psoas; piriformis—myofascial restrictions
**Ergonomics**
Fair

## ASSESSMENT

The patient presents with spondylolisthesis that possibly occurred when she was a gymnast in college. There were trigger points in bilateral psoas; iliacus; quadratus lumborum; and the piriformis. Myofascial restrictions noted in bilateral psoas and piriformis, which is causing decreased hip internal rotation and hip extension is increasing shear force in the lumbar spine secondary to compensatory movement patterns. Spinal extension increases. Core weakness was noted.

### Plan

Self–myofascial release/corrective flexibility/corrective exercises/corrective manual therapy/modalities

### Self–Myofascial Release

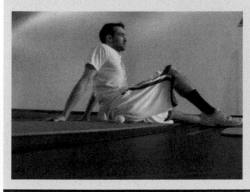

**FIGURE 18.1.** Tennis ball: bilateral piriformis.

## Corrective Flexibility

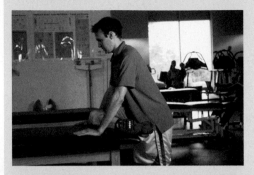

**FIGURE 18.2A.** Static: bilateral piriformis on bench.

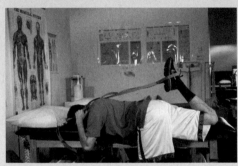

**FIGURE 18.2B.** Active: bilateral rectus femoris/prone.

## Corrective Exercise

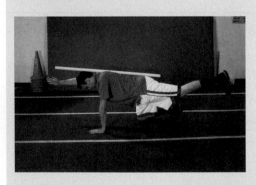

**FIGURE 18.3A.** Quadruped: alternate limb extensions/ with dowel vertical.

(*continued*)

## Corrective Exercise (*continued*)

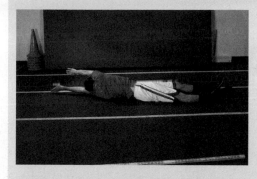

**FIGURE 18.3B.** Rolling: supine to prone arm drive.

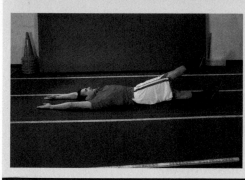

**FIGURE 18.3C.** Rolling: supine to prone leg drive.

## Manual Therapy

1. Warming technique: lumbar erectors; bilateral piriformis
2. Inhibitory technique: bilateral psoas; quadratus lumborum
3. Elongation technique: bilateral piriformis; bilateral psoas
4. Joint mobilizations: bilateral hip internal rotation

## Modalities: prn

## Home Exercise Program

1. Tennis ball: bilateral piriformis
2. Static: piriformis

Orthopedic and Rehabilitation Associates
Orthopedic Street
Omaha, OH
(555) 555-5555
Fax. (666) 666-7777

PATIENT: _Ms. A_
DATE: _2009_

## ORTHOPAEDIC REHABILITATION PRESCRIPTION

*REHAB THERAPIES* ☒ PT ☐ OT ☐ SESSIONS/WK _2_
TOTAL _12_

☒ NEW DIAGNOSIS ☐ RE-EVALUATION ☒ OUTPATIENT

DIAGNOSIS1 _Spondylolisthesis_
  ICD _____

DIAGNOSIS2 _Back pain_
  ICD _____

PREGNANT? ☐ YES ☒ NO    PERTINENTMEDICALHISTORY: _None_

GOALS:
MD/DO: ☒ INCREASE MOBILITY ☒ INCREASE ADL ☒ INCREASE STRENGTH ☒ DECREASE PAIN

PRECAUTIONS: ☐ CARDIAC    MAX-SBP_____ DBP_____ HR_____
ABOVE BASELINE ☐ DIABETES: HYPER/HYPOGLYCEMIA ☐ ORTHOSTASIS
☐ OTHER _____
WEIGHT BEARING: ☐ WBAT ☐ TTWB ☐ NWB
  TO: _____
MODALITIES: ☐ ULTRASOUND TO: _Lumbar paraspinals x 7 min_
      ☐ E-STIM    TO: _Lumbar paraspinals x 7 min B/L_

B/L _____
    ☐ FLUID THERAPY ☐ JOBST ☐ PARAFFIN
  TO: _____
    ☐ ICE    TO: _10 min to lumbara paraspinals_
B/L _____
    ☐ HOTPACKS    TO: _10 min to lumbara paraspinals_
    ☐ EXERCISES ☐ PROM ☐ AAROM ☐ AROM
  TO: _B/L LE_
    ☒ PRE's ☐ ISOMETRICS ☐ ISOKINETICS
  TO: _B/L LE_
    ☐ SLIDEBOARD ☐ PLYOMETRICS ☐ MODIFIED KNEE BEND
☐ STEPUPS
☒ LUMBAR STABILIZATION ☒ WILLIAM's ☐ McKENZIE ☐ CERVICAL EXERCISES
☐ RELAXATION ☐ COORDINATION
MANUAL: ☒ CONTRACT RELAX ☐ CRANIOSACRAL ☒ JONES/C-STRAIN ☒ SOFT
TISSUE MOBILIZATION
    ☒ STRETCHING ☒ MASSAGE ☒ MYOF AS RELEASE ☒ SPRAY/STRETCH
  TO: _LE B/L_
EDUCATION: ☒ MOBILITY: ☐ TRANSFERS ☒ ADL ☒ HEP ☐ ENERGY CONSERV
☐ WORK HARDENING ☒ BIOMECHANICS ☐ 1
HANDED TECHNIQUES
☐ GAIT TRAINING ☐ FINE MOTOR ☐ COORD/BALANCE
OTHER: _____
_____
_____

ADL-ACTIVITIES OF DAILY LIVING    AAROM-ACTIVE/ASSISTIVERANGEOFMOTION   DBP-
DIASTOLIC BLOOD PRESSURE
SBP-SYSTOLIC BLOOD PRESSURE    HR-HEART RATE   HEP-HOME EXERCISE PROGRAM
NWB-NON-WEIGHT BEARING
PRE's-PROGRESSIVE RESISTIVE EXERCISES    WBAT-WEIGHT BEARING AS TOLERATED
ROM-RANGE OF MOTION

The above is medically necessary to decrease debility and achieve ADL independence. Also to:
☒ decrease pain, ☒ improve strength/endurance, ☒ improve balance coordination, ☒ improve gait,
☐ improve transfers,
Other _____

PHYSICIAN'S SIGNATURE _____ DATE _____

# CASE 19

# FACET ARTHROPATHY

**CC:** Back pain

**HPI:** Mr. V is a 64-year-old male with a 3-year history of lower back pain. He says the pain began gradually and without inciting event. The pain is localized to the lower back and does not radiate into his lower extremities. He denies any numbness, tingling, or burning. The pain is described as a dull ache and is 5/10 intensity. He went to his PMD a year ago. He did not get any x-rays taken but was sent for physical therapy. He went to therapy for a few sessions but did not feel it was helping, so he stopped. Since that time, he has been taking Tylenol for the pain. The pain is much worse while standing and walking and better with sitting or resting.

**PMHx:** High cholesterol, BPH

**PSHx:** None

**Meds:** Crestor, Flomax

**Allergies:** NKDA

**Social:** No smoking. One glass of red wine every night.

**ROS:** Noncontributory

## PHYSICAL EXAMINATION

On exam, Mr. V is pleasant and in no acute distress. He looks his stated age. BP: 132/88, P: 70, RR: 14. He has increased pain with trunk extension and no pain with trunk flexion. He has 5/5 strength, 2 + patella and Achilles reflexes, and intact sensation in the bilateral lower extremities. No pathologic reflexes are elicited. He has a negative FABER, slump, and SLR test bilaterally. Tenderness is noted over the bilateral L4-5 paraspinals. There is no bony tenderness elicited. The SI joint is not tender. He has no pain with maximal simultaneous passive hip and knee flexion. Pain is exacerbated by arching his lower back while prone. 2+ distal pulses are palpated bilaterally.

## Impression

Facet arthropathy

## Plan

1. X-ray
2. Physical therapy

# PHYSICAL THERAPY

The patient is a 64-year-old male who presents with lower back pain that started 3 years ago with an insidious onset. The pain is localized to the lower back with no radicular symptoms. The patient had three physical therapy sessions about a year ago and discontinued physical therapy. The patient went to the physician and was referred to physical therapy.

**Scale:** 5/10

**Increase pain:** prolonged walking; prolonged standing

**Decrease pain:** sitting; lying in side line with torso rotation

## Range of Motion

**Lumbar spine**

Flexion: 75% with no pain

Extension: 75% with pain

Left sidebending: 75% with pain

Right sidebending: 75% with pain

Left rotation: 50% no pain

Right rotation: 50% no pain

**Thoracic spine**

T/S rotation left: 50%

T/S rotation right: 50%

T/S flexion: WNL

T/S extension: 75%

**Hip**

Left hip extension: −10 degrees

Right hip extension: −10 degrees

Bilateral prone hip internal rotation: −10 degrees

**Joint play**

L/S 2/6 throughout

**Special tests**

Spurling's + with pain

SLR −

Vasalva −

**Manual muscle testing**
Core: 4/5 throughout
Psoas: 4/5 bilateral
Piriformis: 4/5 bilateral
**Tight tender points/soft tissue restrictions**
Bilateral psoas; iliacus; quadratus lumborum; piriformis—trigger points
Bilateral psoas; piriformis; thoracic spine erectors—myofascial restrictions
**Ergonomics**
Fair

## ASSESSMENT

The patient presents with facet arthropathy. The patient presents with trigger points in bilateral psoas; iliacus; quadratus lumborum; and the piriformis. Myofascial restrictions noted in bilateral psoas; piriformis; and thoracic erectors. There is decreased T/S and hip rotation, which has increased lumbar spine stress and facet wear. Lumbar spine gapping decreases symptoms. Core weakness was noted.

### Plan

Self–myofascial release/corrective flexibility/corrective exercises/corrective manual therapy/modalities

### Self–Myofascial Release

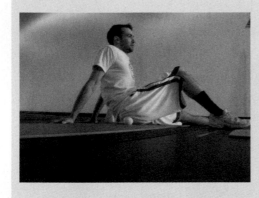

**FIGURE 19.1A.** Tennis ball: bilateral piriformis.

(*continued*)

## Self–Myofascial Release (*continued*)

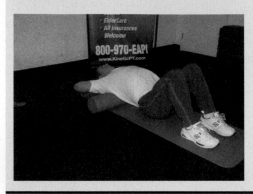

**FIGURE 19.1B.** Foam roll: T/S perpendicular.

## Corrective Flexibility

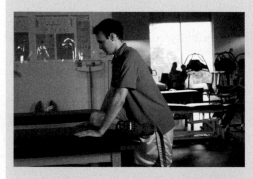

**FIGURE 19.2A.** Static: bilateral piriformis on bench.

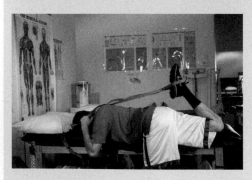

**FIGURE 19.2B.** Static: bilateral rectus femoris/prone.

(*continued*)

## Corrective Flexibility (*continued*)

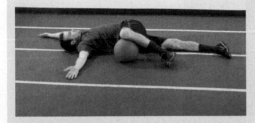

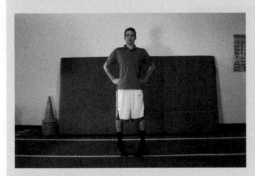

**FIGURE 19.2C.** Active: T/S rotation in side line with pectoralis.

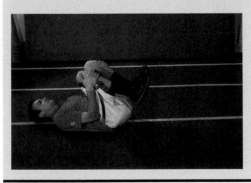

**FIGURE 19.2D.** Active: progressive hip internal rotation.

**FIGURE 19.2E.** Active: double knees to chest.

## Corrective Exercise

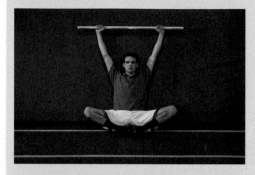

**FIGURE 19.3A.** Wall sit: shoulder extension.

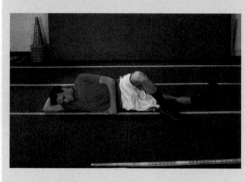

**FIGURE 19.3B.** Side line: hip internal rotation bilateral.

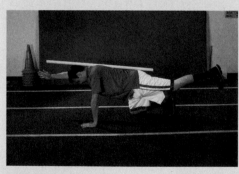

**FIGURE 19.3C.** Quadruped: alternate limb extension with dowel.

## Manual Therapy

1. Warming technique: lumbar erectors; bilateral piriformis
2. Inhibitory technique: bilateral psoas; quadratus lumborum
3. Elongation technique: bilateral piriformis; bilateral psoas
4. Joint mobilizations: bilateral hip internal rotation
5. Joint mobilizations: T/S rotation

## Modalities: prn

## Home Exercise Program

1. Tennis ball: bilateral piriformis
2. Static: piriformis
3. Active: double knee to chest

Orthopedic and Rehabilitation Associates
Orthopedic Street
Omaha, OH
(555) 555-5555
Fax. (666) 666-7777

PATIENT: _Mr. V_
DATE: _2009_

## ORTHOPAEDIC REHABILITATION PRESCRIPTION

| REHAB THERAPIES | ☒ PT | ☐ OT | ☐ SESSIONS/WK _2_ |
| TOTAL _12_ | | | |

☒ NEW DIAGNOSIS    ☐ RE-EVALUATION    ☒ OUTPATIENT

DIAGNOSIS1 _Facet Arthropathy_
 ICD _____

DIAGNOSIS2 _____
 ICD _____

PREGNANT? ☐ YES ☒ NO        PERTINENTMEDICALHISTORY: _None_

GOALS:
MD/DO: ☒ INCREASE MOBILITY ☒ INCREASE ADL ☒ INCREASE STRENGTH ☒ DECREASE PAIN

PRECAUTIONS: ☐ CARDIAC    MAX-SBP_____ DBP_____ HR_____
ABOVE BASELINE    ☐ DIABETES: HYPER/HYPOGLYCEMIA    ☐ ORTHOSTASIS
☐ OTHER _____

WEIGHT BEARING:    ☐ WBAT    ☐ TTWB    ☐ NWB
 TO: _____

MODALITIES: ☐ ULTRASOUND TO: _Lumbar paraspinals x 7 Min_
         ☐ E-STIM      TO: _Lumbar Paraspinals x 7 min_

     ☐ FLUID THERAPY    ☐ JOBST    ☐ PARAFFIN
 TO: _____
     ☐ ICE    TO: _10 min to lumbar paraspinals_

     ☐ HOTPACKS    TO: _10 min to lumbar paraspinals_
     ☐ EXERCISES ☐ PROM ☐ AAROM ☐ AROM
 TO: _B/L LE_
     ☒ PRE's ☐ ISOMETRICS ☐ ISOKINETICS
 TO: _B/L LE_
         ☐ SLIDEBOARD ☐ PLYOMETRICS ☐ MODIFIED KNEE BEND
☐ STEPUPS
☒ LUMBAR STABILIZATION ☒ WILLIAM's ☐ McKENZIE ☐ CERVICAL EXERCISES
☐ RELAXATION ☐ COORDINATION

MANUAL: ☒ CONTRACT RELAX ☐ CRANIOSACRAL ☒ JONES/C-STRAIN ☒ SOFT
TISSUE MOBILIZATION
     ☒ STRETCHING ☒ MASSAGE ☒ MYOF AS RELEASE ☒ SPRAY/STRETCH
 TO: _LE B/L_
EDUCATION: ☒ MOBILITY: ☐ TRANSFERS ☒ ADL ☒ HEP ☐ ENERGY CONSERV
     ☐ WORK HARDENING ☒ BIOMECHANICS ☐ 1
HANDED TECHNIQUES
     ☐ GAIT TRAINING ☐ FINE MOTOR ☐ COORD/BALANCE
OTHER: _____
_____
_____

ADL-ACTIVITIES OF DAILY LIVING    AAROM-ACTIVE/ASSISTIVERANGEOFMOTION   DBP-
DIASTOLIC BLOOD PRESSURE
SBP-SYSTOLIC BLOOD PRESSURE    HR-HEART RATE    HEP-HOME EXERCISE PROGRAM
NWB-NON-WEIGHT BEARING
PRE's-PROGRESSIVE RESISTIVE EXERCISES    WBAT-WEIGHT BEARING AS TOLERATED
ROM-RANGE OF MOTION

The above is medically necessary to decrease debility and achieve ADL independence. Also to:
☒ decrease pain, ☒ improve strength/endurance, ☒ improve balance coordination, ☒ improve gait,
☐ improve transfers,
Other _____

PHYSICIAN'S SIGNATURE _____ DATE _____

# CASE 20

## SACROILIAC JOINT PAIN

**CC:** Back pain

**HPI:** Ms. X is 42 years old and has a history of L3-S1 fusion in 1992 for chronic lower back pain. Following her surgery, she felt 90% better until 3 months ago when her pain returned. The pain is in a slightly different location than before. It is more inferior, in the buttocks. She says the pain is sometimes "sharp" and sometimes "dull." There is no radiation of symptoms. No numbness, tingling, or burning. No weakness. She went to her spine surgeon who took x-rays and confirmed that the hardware was in place. The surgeon felt she was not a surgical candidate and referred her to this office for further evaluation. Her pain is currently 4/10 intensity. She is taking Flexeril and Vicodin prn, which the surgeon gave her. These medications help the pain and allow her to function during the day and to sleep at night. The pain is worse with walking and better with rest.

**PMHx:** None
**PSHx:** None
**Meds:** Flexeril and vicodin
**Allergies:** NKDA
**Social:** No smoking. Social EtOH.
**ROS:** Noncontributory

## PHYSICAL EXAMINATION

On exam, Ms. X is pleasant and in no acute distress. She looks her stated age. BP: 120/76, P: 64, RR: 14. She has minimal pain with trunk flexion and extension. She has 5/5 strength, 2+ patella and Achilles reflexes, and intact sensation in the bilateral lower extremities. No pathologic reflexes are elicited. She has a positive FABER test and her SI joint is tender. She has a negative slump and SLR test bilaterally. There is no tenderness over the paraspinals. There is no bony tenderness elicited. She has no pain with maximal simultaneous passive hip and knee flexion. 2+ distal pulses are palpated bilaterally.

### Impression

SI joint pain

### Plan

**1.** Physical therapy

## PHYSICAL THERAPY

The patient is a 42-year-old female who presents with lower back pain that started 3 months ago with an insidious onset. Past medical history included L3-S1 spinal fusion in 1992 where pain had tingling and numbness down the left leg. No tingling and numbness currently noted. Current symptoms are in a different location. The pain is localized to the lower back with no radicular symptoms. The patient went to the physician and was referred to physical therapy.
**Scale:** 4/10
**Increase pain:** pain is localized and fixed; no movements increase symptoms; constant

### Range of Motion

**Lumbar spine**
Flexion: WNL
Extension: WNL
Left sidebending: WNL
Right sidebending: WNL
Left rotation: WNL
Right rotation: WNL
**Thoracic spine**
T/S rotation left: WNL
T/S rotation right: WNL
T/S flexion: WNL
T/S extension: WNL
**Hip**
Left hip extension: 0 degrees
Right hip extension: –10 degrees

Left hip flexion hip internal rotation: −10 degrees
Left long axis internal rotation: 0
**Joint play**
L/S WNL
Left hip posterior capsule 2/6
**Special tests**
Left leg length discrepancy ¼ in short
Long slt test + left leg lengthened
SLR −
**Manual muscle testing**
Core: 4/5 throughout
Psoas: 3/5 left
Gluteus medius: posterior fibers left 3/5
Tensor fascia latae: left 3/5
**Neurodynamic assessment**
Left side common peroneal nerve restrictions
**Tight tender points/soft tissue restrictions**
Left psoas; iliacus; gluteus medius posterior fibers—trigger points
Left biceps femoris long head—myofascial restrictions
**Ergonomics**
Fair

## ASSESSMENT

The patient presents with left-sided SI joint dysfunction. The patient presents with a functional leg length discrepancy with trigger points in left psoas; iliacus. Myofascial restrictions noted in left biceps femoris long head. The patient also presents with neural adhesions around the common peroneal nerve as shown during neurodynamic assessments and palpating the biceps femoris attachment to the fibular head. Core weakness was noted along with left psoas and posterior gluteus medius.

### Plan

Self–myofascial release/corrective flexibility/corrective exercises/corrective manual therapy/modalities

## Self–Myofascial Release

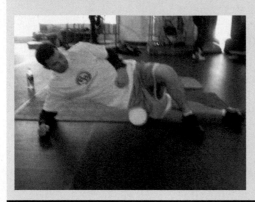

**FIGURE 20.1.** Tennis ball: left gluteus medius posterior fibers; left ITB/TFL.

## Corrective Flexibility

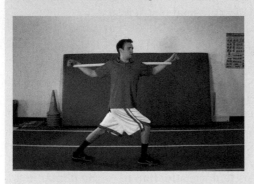

**FIGURE 20.2A.** Static: left-sided psoas in standing.

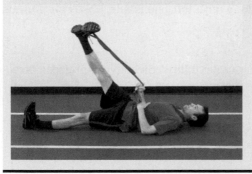

**FIGURE 20.2B.** Neuromobilization: common peroneal nerve left.

## Corrective Exercise

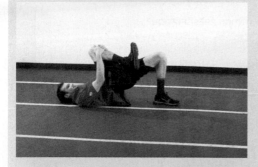

**FIGURE 20.3A.** Bridge: leg lock left side only with knee bent.

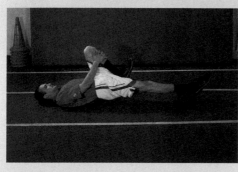

**FIGURE 20.3B.** Bridge: leg lock left side only foam roll under ankle.

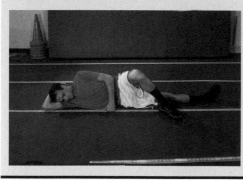

**FIGURE 20.3C.** Side line: hip internal left side only.

## Manual Therapy

1. Warming technique: bilateral gluteus maximus
2. Inhibitory technique: left psoas; posterior gluteus medius
3. Elongation technique: left psoas
4. Neuromobilization: left side common peroneal nerve

## Modalities: prn

## Home Exercise Program

1. Tennis ball: left side ITB/TFL; posterior gluteus medius
2. Static: psoas

Orthopedic and Rehabilitation Associates                    PATIENT: *Ms. X*
Orthopedic Street                                          DATE: *2009*
Omaha, OH
(555) 555-5555
Fax. (666) 666-7777

### ORTHOPAEDIC REHABILITATION PRESCRIPTION

*REHAB THERAPIES*    ☒ PT    ☐ OT    ☐ SESSIONS/WK *2*
TOTAL *12*

☒ NEW DIAGNOSIS    ☐ RE-EVALUATION    ☒ OUTPATIENT

DIAGNOSIS1 *SI Joint Pain*
   ICD _____

DIAGNOSIS2 _____
   ICD _____

PREGNANT? ☐ YES ☒ NO    PERTINENTMEDICALHISTORY: *None*

GOALS:
MD/DO: ☒ INCREASE MOBILITY ☒ INCREASE ADL ☒ INCREASE STRENGTH ☒ DECREASE PAIN

PRECAUTIONS: ☐ CARDIAC    MAX-SBP ____ DBP ____ HR ____
ABOVE BASELINE    ☐ DIABETES: HYPER/HYPOGLYCEMIA ☐ ORTHOSTASIS
☐ OTHER _____
WEIGHT BEARING:    ☐ WBAT    ☐ TTWB    ☐ NWB
TO: _____
MODALITIES: ☐ ULTRASOUND TO: *NO ULTRASOUND*
     ☐ E-STIM    TO: *SI Joint x 7 minutes*

    ☐ FLUID THERAPY    ☐ JOBST    ☐ PARAFFIN
TO: _____
    ☒ ICE    TO: *10 min to SI Joint and paraspinals*

    ☒ HOTPACKS    TO: *10 min to SI Joint and paraspinals*
    ☐ EXERCISES ☐ PROM ☐ AAROM ☐ AROM
TO: *B/L LE*
    ☒ PRE's ☐ ISOMETRICS ☐ ISOKINETICS
TO: *BL L/E*
    ☐ SLIDEBOARD ☐ PLYOMETRICS ☐ MODIFIED KNEE BEND
☐ STEPUPS
☒ LUMBAR STABILIZATION ☐ WILLIAM's ☐ McKENZIE ☐ CERVICAL EXERCISES
☐ RELAXATION ☐ COORDINATION
MANUAL: ☒ CONTRACT RELAX ☐ CRANIOSACRAL ☒ JONES/C-STRAIN ☒ SOFT
TISSUE MOBILIZATION
    ☒ STRETCHING ☒ MASSAGE ☒ MYOF AS RELEASE ☒ SPRAY/STRETCH
TO: *LE B/L Cervical paraspinals*
EDUCATION: ☒ MOBILITY: ☐ TRANSFERS ☒ ADL ☒ HEP ☐ ENERGY CONSERV
☐ WORK HARDENING ☒ BIOMECHANICS ☐ 1
HANDED TECHNIQUES
☐ GAIT TRAINING ☐ FINE MOTOR ☐ COORD/BALANCE
OTHER: _____
_____
_____

ADL-ACTIVITIES OF DAILY LIVING    AAROM-ACTIVE/ASSISTIVERANGEOFMOTION    DBP-
DIASTOLIC BLOOD PRESSURE
SBP-SYSTOLIC BLOOD PRESSURE    HR-HEART RATE    HEP-HOME EXERCISE PROGRAM
NWB-NON-WEIGHT BEARING
PRE's-PROGRESSIVE RESISTIVE EXERCISES    WBAT-WEIGHT BEARING AS TOLERATED
ROM-RANGE OF MOTION

The above is medically necessary to decrease debility and achieve ADL independence. Also to:
☒ decrease pain, ☒ improve strength/endurance, ☒ improve balance coordination, ☒ improve gait,
☐ improve transfers,
Other _____

PHYSICIAN'S SIGNATURE _____ DATE _____

# CASE 21

## SPINAL STENOSIS

**CC:** Back and bilateral lower extremity pain

**HPI:** Mr. B is 68 years old and complains of 4 months of achy lower back pain and radiating "burning" leg pain. The pain radiates through his buttocks, posterior thighs, and into the posterior calves. The right leg is more painful than the left. The lower back pain is constant but the leg pain is intermittent. The back and leg pain are worse with standing and walking. Sitting and bending forward make the pain better. Mr. B used to be an active walker, but in the last 2 months he has to stop repeatedly after just a few blocks of walking because the pain increases too much. He rates the pain as 2/10 at rest, but 6 or 7/10 while walking. This is the first time that he is coming to the doctor for this problem. He has not had any imaging studies of his spine, and he does not take any pain medications. No change in bowel or bladder.

**PMHx:** HTN

**PSHx:** None

**Meds:** Enalapril

**Allergies:** Sulfa gives a rash

**Social:** No smoking. Social EtOH.

**ROS:** Noncontributory

## PHYSICAL EXAMINATION

On exam, Mr. B is pleasant and in no acute distress. He looks his stated age. BP: 134/88, P: 66, RR: 14. He has lower back pain, but not leg pain, with trunk extension but no pain with trunk flexion. He has 5/5 strength, 2+ patella and Achilles reflexes, and intact sensation in the bilateral lower extremities. No pathologic reflexes are elicited. He has a negative FABER test and his SI joint is not tender. He has a positive slump and SLR test bilaterally. There is tenderness over the paraspinals, right worse than left. There is no bony tenderness elicited. He has no pain with maximal simultaneous passive hip and knee flexion. 2+ distal pulses are palpated bilaterally.

### Impression

Spinal stenosis

### Plan

1. X-rays
2. Physical therapy

## PHYSICAL THERAPY

The patient is a 68-year-old male who presents with lower back pain that started 4 months ago. The pain radiates down the posterior aspect of both legs, the right is more painful than the left.

**Scale:** 2/10 at rest, 6–7/10 at most

**Increase pain:** walking; standing >8 minutes; bending backward

**Decrease pain:** sitting; bending forward

### Range of Motion

**Lumbar spine**
Flexion: 75%
Extension: 25% with pain down both legs
Left sidebending: 75%
Right sidebending: 75%
Left rotation: 75%
Right rotation: 75%
**Thoracic spine**
T/S rotation left: 75%
T/S rotation right: 75%
T/S flexion: WNL
T/S extension: 50%
**Hip**
Left hip extension: –5 degrees
Right hip extension: –5 degrees
Bilateral hip flexion hip internal rotation: –10 degrees
**Joint play**
L/S: L1-5 2/6 with reproduction of symptoms

**Special tests**
Bicycle test +
SLR –
**Manual muscle testing**
Core: 4/5 throughout
Psoas: 3/5 bilateral
Quadratus lumborum: 3/5 bilateral
**Neurodynamic assessment**
Tight tender points/soft tissue restrictions:
Bilateral psoas; iliacus; piriformis; quadratus lumborum—trigger points
Bilateral psoas—myofascial restrictions
**Posture**
Increased kyphosis in thoracic spine; increased forward head posture;
decreased lumbar lordosis
**Ergonomics**
Fair

## ASSESSMENT

The patient presents with signs and symptoms consistent with spinal
stenosis. The patient presents with dysfunctional painful movement patterns in lumbar extension. The patient has poor lordotic curvature in the
lumbar spine. Bicycle test was positive. Trigger points in bilateral psoas;
iliacus, piriformis, and quadratus lumborum. Myofascial restrictions
noted in bilateral psoas. Core weakness was noted along with weakness
in bilateral psoas and quadratus lumborum.

### Plan

Self–myofascial release/corrective flexibility/corrective exercises/correc-
tive manual therapy/modalities

### Self–Myofascial Release

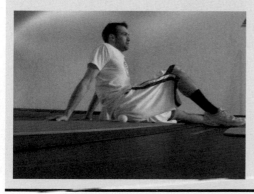

**FIGURE 21.1.** Tennis ball
bilateral piriformis.

## Corrective Flexibility

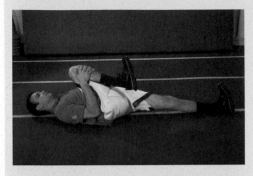

**FIGURE 21.2A.** Active: single knee to chest.

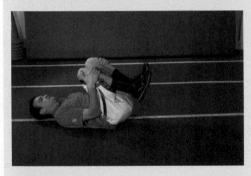

**FIGURE 21.2B.** Active: double knee to chest.

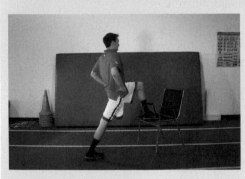

**FIGURE 21.2C.** Active: hip flexor stretch with three directions.

*(continued)*

## Corrective Flexibility (*continued*)

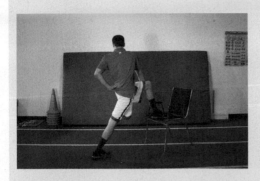

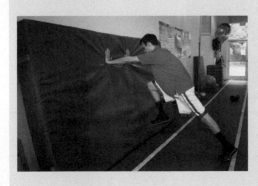

## Corrective Exercise

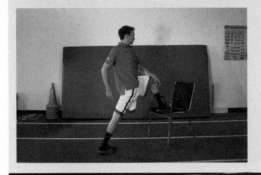

**FIGURE 21.3A.** Wall push knee to chest.

(*continued*)

## Corrective Exercise (*continued*)

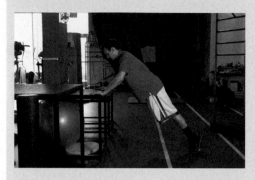

**FIGURE 21.3B.** Push up with an incline.

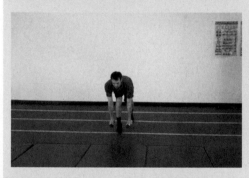

**FIGURE 21.3C.** Lunge: anteriorly with anterior reach down.

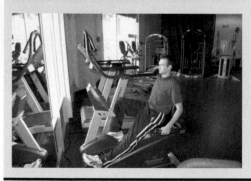

**FIGURE 21.3D.** Bicycle.

## Manual Therapy

1. Warming technique: bilateral gluteus maximus and quadratus lumborum
2. Inhibitory technique: bilateral psoas and quadratus lumborum
3. Elongation technique: bilateral psoas

## Modalities: prn

## Home Exercise Program

1. Tennis ball: bilateral piriformis
2. Active: single knee to chest
3. Active: double knee to chest

Orthopedic and Rehabilitation Associates
Orthopedic Street
Omaha, OH
(555) 555-5555
Fax. (666) 666-7777

PATIENT: _Mr. B_
DATE: _2009_

## ORTHOPAEDIC REHABILITATION PRESCRIPTION

*REHAB THERAPIES*   ☒ PT   ☐ OT   ☐ SESSIONS/WK _2_
TOTAL _12_

☒ NEW DIAGNOSIS   ☐ RE-EVALUATION   ☒ OUTPATIENT

DIAGNOSIS1 _Spinal stenosis_
ICD _____

DIAGNOSIS2 _____
ICD _____

PREGNANT? ☐ YES ☒ NO   PERTINENTMEDICALHISTORY: _None_

GOALS:
MD/DO: ☒ INCREASE MOBILITY ☒ INCREASE ADL ☒ INCREASE STRENGTH ☒ DECREASE PAIN

PRECAUTIONS: ☐ CARDIAC   MAX-SBP ____ DBP ____ HR ____
ABOVE BASELINE   ☐ DIABETES: HYPER/HYPOGLYCEMIA ☐ ORTHOSTASIS
☐ OTHER _____
WEIGHT BEARING: ☐ WBAT ☐ TTWB ☐ NWB
TO: _____
MODALITIES: ☐ ULTRASOUND TO: _B/L lumbar paraspinals x 1 min_
          ☐ E-STIM   TO: _B/L lumbar paraspinals x 1 min_

    ☐ FLUID THERAPY   ☐ JOBST   ☐ PARAFFIN
TO: _____
    ☒ ICE   TO: _10 min to B/L lumbar paraspinals_

    ☒ HOTPACKS   TO: _10 min to B/L lumbar paraspinals_
    ☐ EXERCISES ☐ PROM ☐ AAROM ☐ AROM
TO: _B/L LE_
    ☒ PRE's ☐ ISOMETRICS ☐ ISOKINETICS
TO: _B/L LE_
    ☐ SLIDEBOARD ☐ PLYOMETRICS ☐ MODIFIED KNEE BEND
☐ STEPUPS
☒ LUMBAR STABILIZATION ☐ WILLIAM's ☐ McKENZIE ☐ CERVICAL EXERCISES
☐ RELAXATION ☐ COORDINATION
MANUAL: ☒ CONTRACT RELAX ☐ CRANIOSACRAL ☒ JONES/C-STRAIN ☒ SOFT
TISSUE MOBILIZATION
    ☒ STRETCHING ☒ MASSAGE ☒ MYOF AS RELEASE ☒ SPRAY/STRETCH
    TO: _LE B/L_
EDUCATION: ☒ MOBILITY: ☐ TRANSFERS ☒ ADL ☒ HEP ☐ ENERGY CONSERV
    ☐ WORK HARDENING ☒ BIOMECHANICS ☐ 1
HANDED TECHNIQUES
    ☐ GAIT TRAINING ☐ FINE MOTOR ☐ COORD/BALANCE
OTHER: _____
_____
_____

ADL-ACTIVITIES OF DAILY LIVING   AAROM-ACTIVE/ASSISTIVERANGEOFMOTION   DBP-
DIASTOLIC BLOOD PRESSURE
SBP-SYSTOLIC BLOOD PRESSURE   HR-HEART RATE   HEP-HOME EXERCISE PROGRAM
NWB-NON-WEIGHT BEARING
PRE's-PROGRESSIVE RESISTIVE EXERCISES   WBAT-WEIGHT BEARING AS TOLERATED
ROM-RANGE OF MOTION

The above is medically necessary to decrease debility and achieve ADL independence. Also to:
☒ decrease pain, ☒ improve strength/endurance, ☒ improve balance coordination, ☒ improve gait,
☐ improve transfers,
Other _____

PHYSICIAN'S SIGNATURE _____ DATE _____

# CASE 22

## ACUTE LUMBAR RADICULITIS

**CC:** Back and leg pain

**HPI:** Mr. R is 39 years old and complains of 1 week of back and shooting left leg pain. He says that the pain began when he was wrestling with his 12-year-old son. He bent forward and felt a "searing" pain down the posterior aspect of the left leg, from the buttock to the bottom of the foot. The pain was so bad that he went to the ER. In the ER, he was given a muscle relaxant, Skelaxin, and Vicodin. He has taken these medications as prescribed since the ER visit, but the pain has only gotten minimally better. He has 4/10 left lower back pain that radiates down his leg whenever he "moves wrong." The leg pain is 9/10 intensity. Sitting is much more painful for him than standing. In the morning, the symptoms are worse. He has trouble sleeping at night because of the pain. No change in bowel or bladder. No fevers, chills, night sweats, or recent unintended weight loss. No numbness, tingling, or weakness.

**PMHx:** None

**PSHx:** None

**Meds:** None

**Allergies:** NKDA

**Social:** No smoking. Social EtOH.

**ROS:** Noncontributory

# PHYSICAL EXAMINATION

On exam, Mr. R is pleasant but in apparent moderate distress. BP: 142/88, P: 64, RR: 14. He has significant pain with trunk flexion and at 30 degrees of flexion, the pain begins to radiate down the posterior leg. Trunk extension does not reproduce symptoms. He is able to do single plantar flexion leg raises bilaterally and has 5/5 strength throughout his lower extremities, as well as 2+ patella and Achilles reflexes, and intact sensation in the bilateral lower extremities. No pathologic reflexes are elicited. He has a positive slump test on the left and positive SLR. SLR on the right reproduces symptoms on the left. He has a negative FABER test and his SI joint is not tender. He has tenderness over the left paraspinals. There is no bony tenderness elicited. Passive maximal simultaneous hip and knee flexion is not possible secondary to pain. 2+ distal pulses are palpated bilaterally.

## Impression

Acute lumbar radiculitis secondary to likely L5-S1 disc herniation.

## Plan

1. MRI L-S spine
2. Medrol dose pack
3. C/W Skelaxin and Vicodin prn
4. Physical therapy

# PHYSICAL THERAPY

The patient is a 39-year-old male who presents with shooting pain down his left leg that started × 1 week ago after wrestling with his son. The patient went to the ER secondary to the intensity of the pain. The patient was referred to physical therapy to address symptoms.

**Scale:** 4/10 in low back and 9/10 down the leg

**Increase pain:** sleeping at night; sidebending left; sitting; forward bending; sneezing

**Decrease pain:** lying sideline; lumbar extension

## Range of Motion

**Lumbar spine**
Flexion: 25% with reproduction of symptoms
Extension: 75% but decreases symptoms
Left sidebending: 25% with reproduction of symptoms
Right sidebending: 75%
Left rotation: 75%
Right rotation: 75%

**Thoracic spine**
T/S rotation left: 75%
T/S rotation right: WNL
T/S flexion: WNL
T/S extension: WNL

**Hip**
Left hip extension: –5 degrees
Right hip extension: –5 degrees
**Joint play**
L/S: L1-5 empty end feel
**Special tests**
SLR + left
Well SLR +
Slump test +
**Manual muscle testing**
Core: 3/5 throughout with pain
Psoas: 3/5 bilateral with pain
Quadratus lumborum: 3/5 bilateral with pain
**Neurodynamic assessment**
Left side sciatic
**Tight tender points/soft tissue restrictions**
Bilateral psoas; iliacus; piriformis; quadratus lumborum—trigger points
Bilateral psoas; piriformis—myofascial restrictions
**Posture**
Right lateral shift
**Ergonomics**
Poor

## ASSESSMENT

The patient presents with signs and symptoms consistent with spinal acute lumbar radiculitis secondary to L5-S1 disc herniation. The patient presents with an increase in symptoms with sitting, sneezing, and forward bending. A positive slump test, straight leg raise test, and well leg raise test were noted in the lumbar spine. Trigger points in bilateral psoas; iliacus, piriformis, and quadratus lumborum. Myofascial restrictions noted in bilateral psoas and piriformis. Core weakness was noted along with weakness in bilateral psoas and quadratus lumborum.

### Plan

Self–myofascial release/corrective flexibility/corrective exercises/corrective manual therapy/modalities.

## Self–Myofascial Release

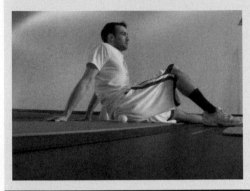

**FIGURE 22.1.** Tennis ball: bilateral piriformis.

## Corrective Flexibility

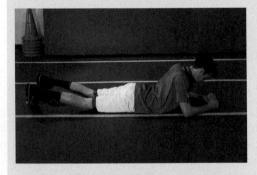

**FIGURE 22.2A.** Static: prone on elbows.

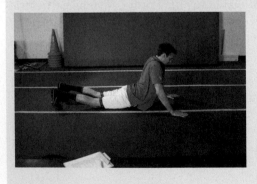

**FIGURE 22.2B.** Active: prone press-up.

(*continued*)

## Corrective Flexibility (*continued*)

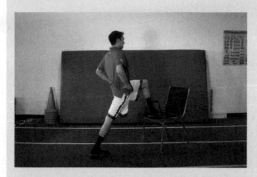

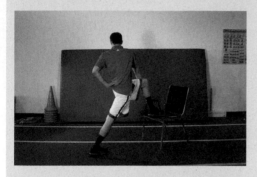

**FIGURE 22.2C.** Active: hip flexor stretch in three directions.

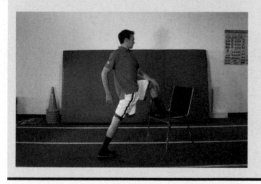

## Corrective Exercise

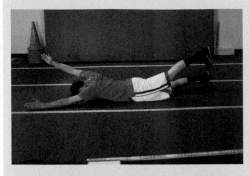

**FIGURE 22.3A.** Prone alternate limb extensions.

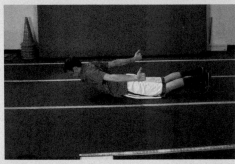

**FIGURE 22.3B.** Prone cobras.

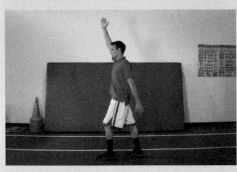

**FIGURE 22.3C.** Walk matrix.

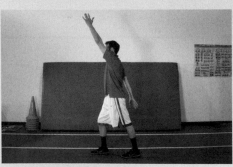

(*continued*)

## Corrective Exercise (*continued*)

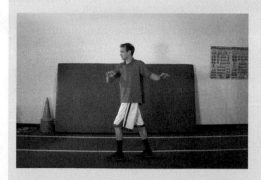

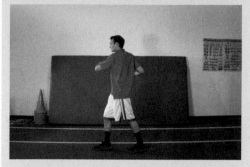

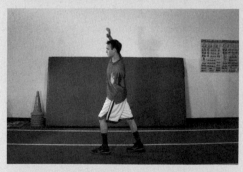

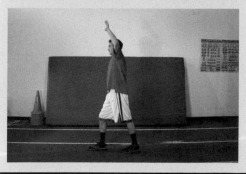

## Manual Therapy

1. Warming technique: bilateral gluteus maximus and quadratus lumborum
2. Inhibitory technique: bilateral psoas and quadratus lumborum
3. Elongation technique: bilateral psoas
4. PA mobilizations to L1-S1
5. PA mobilizations to L1-S1 with prone press-up

## Modalities: prn

## Home Exercise Program

1. Tennis ball: bilateral piriformis
2. Prone press-up

Orthopedic and Rehabilitation Associates
Orthopedic Street
Omaha, OH
(555) 555-5555
Fax. (666) 666-7777

PATIENT: *Mr. R*
DATE: *2009*

## ORTHOPAEDIC REHABILITATION PRESCRIPTION

REHAB THERAPIES ☒ PT ☐ OT ☐ SESSIONS/WK *2*
TOTAL *12*

☒ NEW DIAGNOSIS ☐ RE-EVALUATION ☒ OUTPATIENT

DIAGNOSIS1 *Lumbar Radiculitis*
ICD _____

DIAGNOSIS2 _____
ICD _____

PREGNANT? ☐ YES ☒ NO     PERTINENTMEDICALHISTORY: *None*

GOALS:
MD/DO: ☒ INCREASE MOBILITY ☒ INCREASE ADL ☒ INCREASE STRENGTH ☒ DECREASE PAIN

PRECAUTIONS: ☐ CARDIAC     MAX-SBP ____ DBP ____ HR ____
ABOVE BASELINE     ☐ DIABETES: HYPER/HYPOGLYCEMIA ☐ ORTHOSTASIS
☐ OTHER _____

WEIGHT BEARING: ☐ WBAT ☐ TTWB ☐ NWB
TO: _____

MODALITIES: ☐ ULTRASOUND TO: *NO ULTRASOUND*
☐ E-STIM     TO: *lumbar paraspinals x 7 min*

☐ FLUID THERAPY ☐ JOBST ☐ PARAFFIN
TO: _____
☒ ICE     TO: *10 min to lumbar paraspinals*

☒ HOTPACKS     TO: *10 min to lumbar paraspinals*
☐ EXERCISES ☐ PROM ☐ AAROM ☐ AROM
TO: *B/L LE*
☒ PRE's ☐ ISOMETRICS ☐ ISOKINETICS
TO: *B/L LE*
☐ SLIDEBOARD ☐ PLYOMETRICS ☐ MODIFIED KNEE BEND
☐ STEPUPS
☒ LUMBAR STABILIZATION ☐ WILLIAM's ☒ McKENZIE ☐ CERVICAL EXERCISES
☐ RELAXATION ☐ COORDINATION

MANUAL: ☒ CONTRACT RELAX ☐ CRANIOSACRAL ☒ JONES/C-STRAIN ☒ SOFT
TISSUE MOBILIZATION
☒ STRETCHING ☒ MASSAGE ☒ MYOF AS RELEASE ☒ SPRAY/STRETCH
TO: *LE B/L*

EDUCATION: ☒ MOBILITY: ☐ TRANSFERS ☒ ADL ☒ HEP ☐ ENERGY CONSERV
☐ WORK HARDENING ☒ BIOMECHANICS ☐ 1
HANDED TECHNIQUES
☐ GAIT TRAINING ☐ FINE MOTOR ☐ COORD/BALANCE
OTHER: _____
_____
_____

ADL-ACTIVITIES OF DAILY LIVING     AAROM-ACTIVE/ASSISTIVERANGEOFMOTION     DBP-
DIASTOLIC BLOOD PRESSURE
SBP-SYSTOLIC BLOOD PRESSURE     HR-HEART RATE     HEP-HOME EXERCISE PROGRAM
NWB-NON-WEIGHT BEARING
PRE's-PROGRESSIVE RESISTIVE EXERCISES     WBAT-WEIGHT BEARING AS TOLERATED
ROM-RANGE OF MOTION

The above is medically necessary to decrease debility and achieve ADL independence. Also to:
☒ decrease pain, ☒ improve strength/endurance, ☒ improve balance coordination, ☒ improve gait,
☐ improve transfers,
Other _____

PHYSICIAN'S SIGNATURE _____ DATE _____

# CASE 23

# LUMBAR RADICULOPATHY

**CC:** Leg pain and weakness

**HPI:** Mr. H is 54 years old and complains of pain, numbness, and general weakness in his right leg. He says the pain began about 8 months ago. The pain began in the lower back and then started shooting down the lateral aspect of the thigh and lower leg. Four months ago, the left lateral lower leg and left big toe became numb. He also complains of tingling in this same distribution. "The whole leg just feels weak," he says. No falls while walking. The symptoms are worse when going for a long walk and better with sitting and rest. The pain in the lower back is 3/10, and the pain that shoots down the leg is 5/10. He went to his PMD 7 months ago who took x-rays and told him he has "arthritis." He was sent to physical therapy for 4 weeks but did not notice any improvement. He has not had any MRIs or injections. Mr. H has taken Advil prn, which has not helped. He says the pain is not as bothersome to him as the numbness and sense of weakness. No change in bowel or bladder.

**PMHx:** BPH

**PSHx:** None

**Meds:** Flomax, Advil prn

**Allergies:** NKDA

**Social:** No smoking. Social EtOH.

**ROS:** Noncontributory

# PHYSICAL EXAMINATION

On exam, Mr. H is pleasant and in no acute distress. He looks his stated age. BP: 128/66, P: 66, RR: 14. Trunk extension increases the pain. Trunk flexion does not reproduce any pain. He has 5/5 strength in his lower extremities bilaterally, except that he has 4/5 strength in his left ankle dorsiflexor and 4–/5 left EHL strength. Sensation is intact except that decreased sensation is noted over the dorsal aspect of the left first digit and lower lateral leg. He has 2+ patella and Achilles reflexes. No pathologic reflexes are elicited. He has a positive slump and SLR test on the left. He has a negative FABER test and his SI joint is not tender. He has tenderness over the bilateral paraspinals. There is no bony tenderness elicited. Passive maximal simultaneous hip and knee flexion does not reproduce pain. 2+ distal pulses are palpated bilaterally.

## Impression

Lumbar radiculopathy secondary to spinal stenosis

## Plan

1. MRI L-S spine
2. Physical therapy

# PHYSICAL THERAPY

The patient is a 54-year-old male who presents with pain, numbness, and general weakness in his right leg. The symptoms started 8 months ago. The symptoms travel down the lateral aspect of the thigh and lower leg. The patient was referred to physical therapy to address symptoms.

**Scale:** 3/10 in low back and 5/10 down the leg
**Increase pain:** sleeping at night; long walks; spinal extension;
**Decrease pain:** sitting; rest

## Range of Motion

**Lumbar spine**
Flexion: 100%
Extension: 50% with reproduction of symptoms
Left sidebending: 75%
Right sidebending: 50% with reproduction of symptoms
Left rotation: 100%
Right rotation: 100%
**Thoracic spine**
T/S rotation left: WNL
T/S rotation right: WNL
T/S flexion: WNL
T/S extension: WNL
**Hip**
Left hip extension: WNL
Right hip extension: WNL

**Joint play**
L/S: L3-4 PA joint plays reproduced symptoms
**Special tests**
SLR + right
Spurling's + right
Slump test + right
**Manual muscle testing**
Core: 3/5 throughout with pain
Psoas: 3/5 right with pain
Quadratus lumborum: 3/5 right with pain
**Neurodynamic assessment**
Right side sciatic
**Tight tender points/soft tissue restrictions**
Bilateral psoas; iliacus; piriformis; quadratus lumborum—trigger points
Bilateral psoas; piriformis; quadratus lumborum right—myofascial restrictions
**Ergonomics:** poor

## ASSESSMENT

The patient presents with signs and symptoms consistent with lumbar radiculopathy. The patient presents with an increase in symptoms with walking, prolonged standing, and lumbar extension. A positive slump test, straight leg raise test, and Spurling test were noted on the right side. Trigger points in bilateral psoas; iliacus, piriformis, and quadratus lumborum. Myofascial restrictions noted in right psoas and piriformis. Core weakness was noted along with weakness in right psoas and quadratus lumborum.

### Plan

Self–myofascial release/corrective flexibility/corrective exercises/corrective manual therapy/modalities

## Self–Myofascial Release

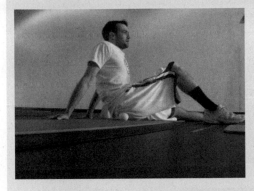

**FIGURE 23.1A.** Tennis ball: bilateral piriformis.

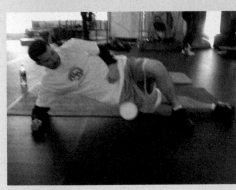

**FIGURE 23.1B.** Foam roll: ITB.

## Corrective Flexibility

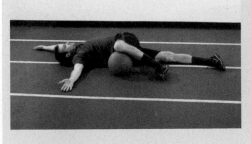

**FIGURE 23.2A.** Static: quadratus lumborum left sideline with right L/S rotation.

*(continued)*

## Corrective Flexibility (*continued*)

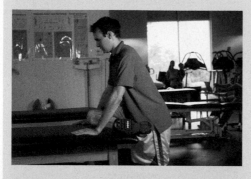

**FIGURE 23.2B.** Static: piriformis bilaterally foot on bench.

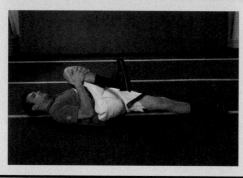

**FIGURE 23.2C.** Active: single knee to chest bilateral.

## Corrective Exercise

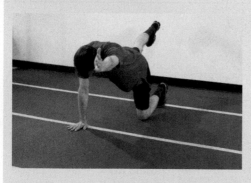

**FIGURE 23.3A.** Quadruped alternate limb extensions.

(*continued*)

## Corrective Exercise (*continued*)

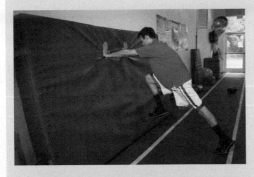

**FIGURE 23.3B.** Wall push with knee to chest.

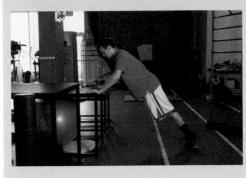

**FIGURE 23.3C.** Push up incline.

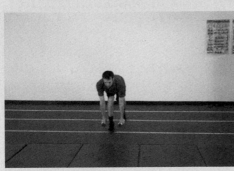

**FIGURE 23.3D.** Split stance anterior reach down.

## Manual Therapy

1. Warming technique: bilateral gluteus maximus and quadratus lumborum
2. Inhibitory technique: right psoas and quadratus lumborum
3. Elongation technique: right quadratus lumborum in left sideline

## Modalities: prn

## Home Exercise Program

1. Tennis ball: bilateral piriformis
2. Static: quadratus lumborum stretch in left sideline with right L/S rotation

Orthopedic and Rehabilitation Associates
Orthopedic Street
Omaha, OH
(555) 555-5555
Fax. (666) 666-7777

PATIENT. _M.R. H_
DATE: _2009_

## ORTHOPAEDIC REHABILITATION PRESCRIPTION

REHAB THERAPIES ☒ PT ☐ OT ☐ SESSIONS/WK _2_
TOTAL _12_

☒ NEW DIAGNOSIS   ☐ RE-EVALUATION   ☒ OUTPATIENT

DIAGNOSIS1 _Lumbar Radiculopathy_
  ICD _____

DIAGNOSIS2 _____
  ICD _____

PREGNANT? ☐ YES ☐ NO      PERTINENT MEDICAL HISTORY: _None_

GOALS:
MD/DO: ☒ INCREASE MOBILITY ☒ INCREASE ADL ☒ INCREASE STRENGTH ☒ DECREASE PAIN

PRECAUTIONS: ☐ CARDIAC    MAX-SBP _____ DBP _____ HR _____
ABOVE BASELINE   ☐ DIABETES: HYPER/HYPOGLYCEMIA ☐ ORTHOSTASIS
☐ OTHER _____

WEIGHT BEARING:   ☐ WBAT   ☐ TTWB   ☐ NWB
  TO: _____

MODALITIES: ☐ ULTRASOUND TO: _NO ULTRASOUND_
        ☐ E-STIM    TO: _lumbar paraspinals x 7 minutes_

     ☐ FLUID THERAPY    ☐ JOBST    ☐ PARAFFIN
  TO: _____
     ☒ ICE    TO: _10 min to lumbar paraspinals_

     ☒ HOTPACKS    TO: _10 min to lumbar paraspinals_
     ☐ EXERCISES  ☐ PROM  ☐ AAROM  ☐ AROM
  TO: _BL L/E_
     ☒ PRE's   ☐ ISOMETRICS   ☐ ISOKINETICS
  TO: _BL L/E_
        ☐ SLIDEBOARD  ☐ PLYOMETRICS  ☐ MODIFIED KNEE BEND
☐ STEP UPS
☒ LUMBAR STABILIZATION ☒ WILLIAM's ☐ McKENZIE ☐ CERVICAL EXERCISES
☐ RELAXATION  ☐ COORDINATION
MANUAL: ☒ CONTRACT RELAX ☐ CRANIOSACRAL ☒ JONES/C-STRAIN ☒ SOFT
TISSUE MOBILIZATION
     ☒ STRETCHING ☒ MASSAGE ☒ MYOF AS RELEASE ☒ SPRAY/STRETCH
  TO: _LE B/L_
EDUCATION: ☒ MOBILITY: ☐ TRANSFERS ☒ ADL ☒ HEP ☐ ENERGY CONSERV
☐ WORK HARDENING ☒ BIOMECHANICS ☐ 1
HANDED TECHNIQUES
☐ GAIT TRAINING ☐ FINE MOTOR ☐ COORD/BALANCE
OTHER: _____
_____
_____

ADL-ACTIVITIES OF DAILY LIVING   AAROM-ACTIVE/ASSISTIVE RANGE OF MOTION   DBP-
DIASTOLIC BLOOD PRESSURE
SBP-SYSTOLIC BLOOD PRESSURE   HR-HEART RATE   HEP-HOME EXERCISE PROGRAM
NWB-NON-WEIGHT BEARING
PRE's-PROGRESSIVE RESISTIVE EXERCISES   WBAT-WEIGHT BEARING AS TOLERATED
ROM-RANGE OF MOTION

The above is medically necessary to decrease debility and achieve ADL independence. Also to:
☒ decrease pain, ☒ improve strength/endurance, ☒ improve balance coordination, ☒ improve gait,
☐ improve transfers,
Other _____

PHYSICIAN'S SIGNATURE _____ DATE _____

# PART **7**

## THIGH PAIN

# CASE 24

# HAMSTRING STRAIN

**CC:** "I pulled my hamstring."

**HPI:** Mr. C is 24 years old and was playing flag football with his friends 1 week ago when he felt something "pull" in his left hamstring. He stopped playing and has been resting and icing it over the last week. He did not notice any significant bruising or swelling. The pain is a little better but he is still unable to run. He wants to make sure that nothing is "torn" and he wants to get back to sport as soon as possible. Denies any back pain. No radiating symptoms. No numbness, tingling, or burning. The pain is in the proximal posterior thigh. At rest there is 1/10 pain, but walking or trying to run increases the pain quickly to 5/10 or higher if he tries to push through it.

**PMHx:** None
**PSHx:** None
**Meds:** None
**Allergies:** NKDA
**Social:** No tobacco. Social EtOH
**ROS:** Noncontributory

## PHYSICAL EXAMINATION

On exam, Mr. C is a well-developed male who looks his stated age. BP: 116/80, P: 64, RR: 14. He is able to toe and heel walk. Trunk flexion creates a pulling sensation that is painful in his left hamstring. Trunk

**183**

extension is not painful. He has a negative SLR and slump test bilaterally. He has 5/5 strength in his bilateral lower extremities, but the exam is limited because left knee flexion and left hip extension could not be fully tested secondary to pain. He has full passive range of motion of his lower extremities bilaterally. No swelling or ecchymosis is present. He has intact sensation, and 2+ patella and Achilles reflexes bilaterally. His left hamstring is tender near its insertion at the ischial tuberosity. 2+ distal pulses are palpated bilaterally.

## Impression

Left hamstring strain

## Plan

1. Physical therapy

# PHYSICAL THERAPY

The patient is a 24-year-old male who presents with left hamstring pain that started while playing flag football × 1 week ago. The patient went to his physician who referred him to physical therapy to treat a proximal hamstring strain.
**Scale:** 1/10 at rest; 5/10
**Increase pain:** walking; climbing stairs; walking up hill; transitioning from sit to stand
**Decrease pain:** sitting; rest

## Range of Motion

**Lumbar spine**
Flexion: 50% with pain left proximal hamstring
Extension: WNL
Left sidebending: WNL
Right sidebending: WNL
Left rotation: WNL
Right rotation: WNL
**Hip**
Left hip extension: WNL
Right hip extension: WNL
Left hip flexion with knee bent: 100 degrees with pain
Right hip flexion with knee bent: WNL
Left hip flexion with knee extension: 30 degrees with pain
Right hip flexion with knee extension: WNL
**Joint play**
WNL
**Special tests**
SLR—left but pain to 30 degrees
**Manual muscle testing**
Core: 3/5 throughout
Psoas: 3/5 left

Piriformis: 3/5 left
Proximal hamstring: 3/5 with pain
**Neurodynamic assessment**
WNL
**Tight tender points/soft tissue restrictions**
Left psoas; iliacus; piriformis; proximal hamstring—trigger points
**Posture**
WNL
**Ergonomics**
WNL

## ASSESSMENT

The patient presents with signs and symptoms consistent with a proximal hamstring strain. The patient presents with an increase in symptoms with walking, climbing stairs, walking up hill, and transitioning from sit to stand position. Trigger points in left psoas; iliacus, piriformis, and proximal hamstring. Core weakness was noted along with weakness in left psoas and proximal hamstring.

### Plan

Self–myofascial release/corrective flexibility/corrective exercises/corrective manual therapy/modalities

### Self–Myofascial Release

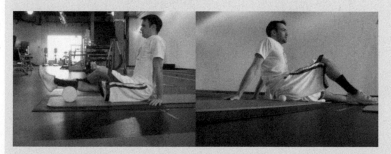

**FIGURE 24.1A.** Tennis ball: left piriformis and left gatroc.

(*continued*)

## Self–Myofascial Release (*continued*)

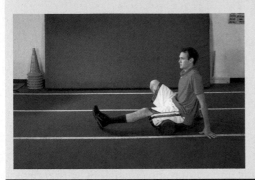

**FIGURE 24.1B.** Foam roll: left hamstring.

## Corrective Flexibility

Early stretching to the hamstring is not recommended. Start introducing low intensity stretching in the second week of rehabilitation.

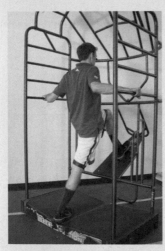

**FIGURE 24.2A.** Active: bilateral psoas.

(*continued*)

## Corrective Exercise

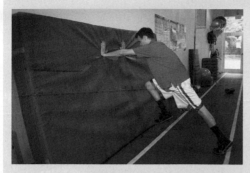

**FIGURE 24.2B.** Wall push with knee to chest.

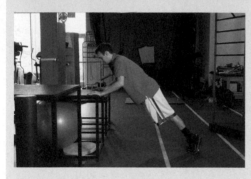

**FIGURE 24.2C.** Push up incline.

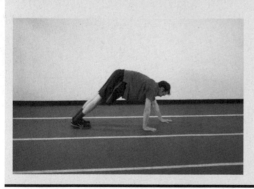

**FIGURE 24.2D.** Walkouts within a painless range.

## Manual Therapy

1. Warming technique: bilateral lumbar erector spinae left hamstring; piriformis; and gastroc
2. Inhibitory technique: left hamstring; piriformis; and gastroc
3. Activation technique: left proximal proximal rectus femoris

## Modalities

1. Ice

## Home Exercise Program

1. Tennis ball: left piriformis, hamstring, and gastroc
2. Ice: prn

Orthopedic and Rehabilitation Associates
Orthopedic Street
Omaha, OH
(555) 555-5555
Fax. (666) 666-7777

PATIENT: _Mr. C_
DATE: _2009_

## ORTHOPAEDIC REHABILITATION PRESCRIPTION

_REHAB THERAPIES_  ☒ PT  ☐ OT  ☐ SESSIONS/WK _2_
TOTAL _12_

☒ NEW DIAGNOSIS  ☐ RE-EVALUATION  ☒ OUTPATIENT

DIAGNOSIS1 _Left Hamstring strain_
  ICD _____

DIAGNOSIS2 _____
  ICD _____

PREGNANT? ☐ YES  ☒ NO    PERTINENTMEDICALHISTORY: _None_

GOALS:
MD/DO: ☒ INCREASE MOBILITY  ☒ INCREASE ADL  ☒ INCREASE STRENGTH  ☒ DECREASE PAIN

PRECAUTIONS: ☐ CARDIAC    MAX-SBP_____ DBP_____ HR_____
ABOVE BASELINE  ☐ DIABETES: HYPER/HYPOGLYCEMIA  ☐ ORTHOSTASIS
☐ OTHER _____
WEIGHT BEARING:  ☐ WBAT  ☐ TTWB  ☐ NWB
  TO: ____
MODALITIES: ☐ ULTRASOUND TO: _Left thigh x 1 min_
       ☐ E-STIM    TO: _Left thigh hand x 1 min B/L_

    ☐ FLUID THERAPY    ☐ JOBST    ☐ PARAFFIN
  TO: _____
    ☐ ICE    TO: _10 min to L thigh_

    ☐ HOTPACKS    TO: _10 min to L thigh_
    ☐ EXERCISES  ☐ PROM  ☐ AAROM  ☐ AROM
  TO: _B/L LE_
    ☒ PRE's  ☐ ISOMETRICS  ☐ ISOKINETICS
  TO: _B/L LE_
    ☐ SLIDEBOARD  ☐ PLYOMETRICS  ☐ MODIFIED KNEE BEND
☒ STEPUPS
☒ LUMBAR STABILIZATION  ☐ WILLIAM's  ☐ McKENZIE  ☐ CERVICAL EXERCISES
☐ RELAXATION  ☐ COORDINATION
MANUAL: ☒ CONTRACT RELAX  ☐ CRANIOSACRAL  ☒ JONES/C-STRAIN  ☒ SOFT
TISSUE MOBILIZATION
    ☒ STRETCHING  ☒ MASSAGE  ☒ MYOF AS RELEASE  ☒ SPRAY/STRETCH
  TO: _LE B/L_
EDUCATION: ☒ MOBILITY:  ☐ TRANSFERS  ☒ ADL  ☒ HEP  ☐ ENERGY CONSERV
    ☐ WORK HARDENING  ☒ BIOMECHANICS  ☐ 1
HANDED TECHNIQUES
    ☐ GAIT TRAINING  ☐ FINE MOTOR  ☐ COORD/BALANCE
OTHER: _____
_____
_____

ADL-ACTIVITIES OF DAILY LIVING    AAROM-ACTIVE/ASSISTIVERANGEOFMOTION  DBP-
DIASTOLIC BLOOD PRESSURE
SBP-SYSTOLIC BLOOD PRESSURE    HR-HEART RATE    HEP-HOME EXERCISE PROGRAM
NWB-NON-WEIGHT BEARING
PRE's-PROGRESSIVE RESISTIVE EXERCISES    WBAT-WEIGHT BEARING AS TOLERATED
ROM-RANGE OF MOTION

The above is medically necessary to decrease debility and achieve ADL independence. Also to:
☒ decrease pain, ☒ improve strength/endurance, ☒ improve balance coordination, ☒ improve gait,
☒ improve transfers,
Other _____

PHYSICIAN'S SIGNATURE _____ DATE _____

# CASE 25

# QUADRICEPS STRAIN

**CC:** "I pulled my thigh muscle."

**HPI:** Ms. K is 20 years old and was playing softball 1 week ago when she felt something "pull" in her left thigh muscle. She stopped playing and has been resting and icing it over the last week. She did not notice any significant bruising or swelling. The pain is a little better but she is still unable to run. She wants to make sure that nothing is "torn" and wants to return to sport as soon as possible. Denies any back pain. No radiating symptoms. No numbness, tingling, or burning. The pain is in the proximal anterior thigh. At rest there is 3/10 pain, but walking or trying to run increases the pain quickly to 5/10 or higher if she tries to push through it.

**PMHx:** None

**PSHx:** None

**Meds:** None

**Allergies:** NKDA

**Social:** She smokes 1 ppd. Social EtOH

**ROS:** Noncontributory

## PHYSICAL EXAMINATION

On exam, Ms. K is a well-developed female who looks her stated age. BP: 110/70, P: 66, RR: 14. She is able to toe and heel walk. Trunk flexion and extension are not painful. She has a negative SLR and slump test bilaterally. She has 5/5 strength in his bilateral lower extremities, but the exam is limited because left knee extension and hip flexion could not be fully tested secondary to pain. She has full passive range of motion of her lower extremities bilaterally, except that knee flexion is limited to 120 degrees secondary to pain. She has a positive Thomas test on the left. No swelling or ecchymosis is present. She has intact sensation, and 2+ patella and Achilles reflexes bilaterally. Her left quadriceps are tender along the proximal portion. 2+ distal pulses are palpated bilaterally.

## Impression

Left quadriceps strain.

## Plan

1. Physical therapy
2. Counseled to quit smoking. Educated as to multiple health risks of continuing.

# PHYSICAL THERAPY

The patient is a 20-year-old female who presents with left anterior thigh pain that started while playing softball × 1 week ago. The patient went to the physician who referred her to physical therapy to treat left quadriceps strain.

**Scale:** 3/10 at rest; 5/10 at most
**Increase pain:** walking; climbing stairs; running; taking a long stride
**Decrease pain:** sitting; rest

## Range of Motion

**Lumbar spine**
Flexion: WNL
Extension: WNL
Left sidebending: WNL
Right sidebending: WNL
Left rotation: WNL
Right rotation: WNL
**Hip**
Left hip extension: –10 degrees with pain
Right hip extension: WNL
Left hip flexion with knee bent: 120 degrees with pain
Right hip flexion with knee bent: WNL
**Joint play**
WNL
**Special tests**
Thomas + left
**Manual muscle testing**
Core: 3/5 throughout
Psoas: 3/5 left with pain
Rectus femoris: 3/5 left with pain

**Neurodynamic assessment**
WNL
**Tight tender points/soft tissue restrictions**
Left psoas; iliacus; proximal rectus femoris—trigger points
Left psoas; iliacus—soft tissue restrictions
**Posture**
WNL
**Ergonomics**
WNL

## ASSESSMENT

The patient presents with signs and symptoms consistent with a proximal rectus femoris strain. The patient presents with an increase in symptoms with walking, climbing stairs, taking a long stride, and pushing off to run. Trigger points in left psoas; iliacus, and rectus femoris. Soft tissue restrictions noted in left psoas and iliacus. Core weakness was noted along with weakness in left psoas and rectus femoris.

### Plan

Self–myofascial release/corrective flexibility/corrective exercises/corrective manual therapy/modalities

### Self–Myofascial Release

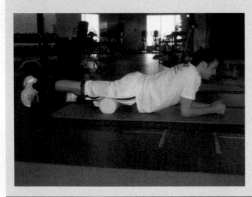

**FIGURE 25.1.** Tennis ball: left rectus femoris.

## Corrective Flexibility

Early stretching to the rectus femoris is not recommended. Start introducing low intensity stretching in the second week of rehabilitation.

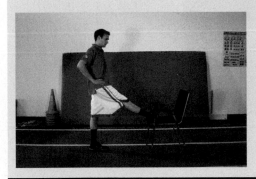

**FIGURE 25.2.** Active: bilateral hamstring.

## Corrective Exercise

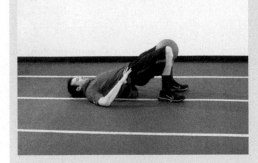

**FIGURE 25.3A.** Bridge: two legs.

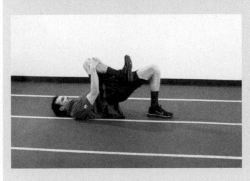

**FIGURE 25.3B.** Bridge: leg lock with knee bent.

*(continued)*

## Corrective Exercise (*continued*)

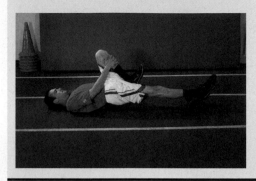

**FIGURE 25.3C.** Bridge: leg lock with knee straight on foam roll.

### Manual Therapy

1. Warming technique: left rectus femoris
2. Inhibitory technique: left rectus femoris, psoas, and iliacus
3. Activation technique: left rectus femoris
4. Elongation technique: left psoas and iliacus

### Modalities

1. Ice

### Home Exercise Program

1. Tennis ball: left rectus femoris
2. Ice: prn

Orthopedic and Rehabilitation Associates
Orthopedic Street
Omaha, OH
(555) 555-5555
Fax. (666) 666-7777

PATIENT: *Ms. K*
DATE: *2009*

## ORTHOPAEDIC REHABILITATION PRESCRIPTION

*REHAB THERAPIES*  ☒ PT    ☐ OT    ☐ SESSIONS/WK *2*
TOTAL *2*

☒ NEW DIAGNOSIS    ☐ RE-EVALUATION    ☒ OUTPATIENT

DIAGNOSIS1 *Left Quadriceps Strain*
　ICD

DIAGNOSIS2
　ICD

PREGNANT? ☐ YES  ☒ NO    PERTINENTMEDICALHISTORY: *None*

GOALS:
MD/DO: ☒ INCREASE MOBILITY ☒ INCREASE ADL ☒ INCREASE STRENGTH ☒ DECREASE PAIN

PRECAUTIONS: ☐ CARDIAC    MAX-SBP____ DBP____ HR____
ABOVE BASELINE    ☐ DIABETES: HYPER/HYPOGLYCEMIA ☐ ORTHOSTASIS
☐ OTHER
WEIGHT BEARING: ☐ WBAT    ☐ TTWB    ☐ NWB
　TO:
MODALITIES: ☐ ULTRASOUND TO: *Left thigh x 1 min*
　　　　　☐ E-STIM    TO: *Left thigh hand x 1 min B/L*

　　　☐ FLUID THERAPY    ☐ JOBST    ☐ PARAFFIN
　TO:
　　　☐ ICE    TO: *10 min to L thigh*

　　　☐ HOTPACKS    TO: *10 min to L thigh*
　　　☐ EXERCISES ☐ PROM ☐ AAROM ☐ AROM
TO: *B/L LE*
　　　☒ PRE's ☐ ISOMETRICS ☐ ISOKINETICS
TO: *B/L LE*
　　　☐ SLIDEBOARD ☐ PLYOMETRICS ☐ MODIFIED KNEE BEND
☐ STEPUPS
☒ LUMBAR STABILIZATION ☐ WILLIAM's ☐ McKENZIE ☐ CERVICAL EXERCISES
☐ RELAXATION ☐ COORDINATION
MANUAL: ☒ CONTRACT RELAX ☐ CRANIOSACRAL ☒ JONES/C-STRAIN ☒ SOFT
TISSUE MOBILIZATION
　　　☒ STRETCHING ☒ MASSAGE ☒ MYOF AS RELEASE ☒ SPRAY/STRETCH
　TO: *LE B/L*
EDUCATION: ☒ MOBILITY: ☐ TRANSFERS ☒ ADL ☒ HEP ☐ ENERGY CONSERV
☐ WORK HARDENING ☒ BIOMECHANICS ☐ 1
HANDED TECHNIQUES
☐ GAIT TRAINING ☐ FINE MOTOR ☐ COORD/BALANCE
OTHER:

ADL-ACTIVITIES OF DAILY LIVING    AAROM-ACTIVE/ASSISTIVERANGEOFMOTION    DBP-
DIASTOLIC BLOOD PRESSURE
SBP-SYSTOLIC BLOOD PRESSURE    HR-HEART RATE    HEP-HOME EXERCISE PROGRAM
NWB-NON-WEIGHT BEARING
PRE's-PROGRESSIVE RESISTIVE EXERCISES    WBAT-WEIGHT BEARING AS TOLERATED
ROM-RANGE OF MOTION

The above is medically necessary to decrease debility and achieve ADL independence. Also to:
☒ decrease pain, ☒ improve strength/endurance, ☒ improve balance coordination, ☒ improve gait,
☒ improve transfers,
Other

PHYSICIAN'S SIGNATURE _____ DATE _____

# PART 8

## KNEE PAIN

# CASE 26

# MENISCUS TEAR

**HPI:** Mr. O is 32 years old and was playing soccer 2 weeks ago when he felt a sudden pain in his right medial knee as he made a cutting movement. He did not hear a "pop" and there was no swelling. He sat out the rest of the game and the pain has not gone away in the subsequent 2 weeks. He has been resting and icing it. No locking, catching, or giving way of the knee. The pain is 5/10 intensity and feels "very stiff and tight." Mr. O is concerned that the pain has persisted for so long and wants to return to sport. No numbness, tingling, or burning.

**PMHx:** None
**PSHx:** None
**Meds:** None
**Allergies:** NKDA
**Social:** No tobacco. Social EtOH
**ROS:** Noncontributory

## PHYSICAL EXAMINATION

On exam, Mr. O is a well-developed male who looks his stated age. BP: 126/70, P: 66, RR: 14. He has 5/5 strength, intact sensation, and 2+ patella and Achilles reflexes in his bilateral lower extremities. Negative J-sign bilaterally. No swelling or ecchymosis is present. In the right knee he has medial joint line tenderness. No peripatellar tenderness. No crepitus. No instability is noted. McMurray's is positive on the right. Apley compression test is positive on the right. The left knee is within normal limits. 2+ distal pulses are palpated bilaterally.

## Impression

Right knee meniscus tear

**Plan**

1. MRI right knee
2. Physical therapy

# PHYSICAL THERAPY

The patient is a 32-year-old male who presents with right knee pain that started × 2 weeks ago while playing soccer. The patient was referred to physical therapy with a diagnosis of right meniscus tear.

**Scale:** 5/10 complaints of stiffness

**Increase pain:** walking; climbing stairs; first thing in the morning; prolonged sit to stand

**Decrease pain:** sitting; rest

## Range of Motion

**Hip**

Left hip extension: WNL

Right hip extension: −10 degrees

Left hip flexion with knee bent: WNL

Right hip flexion with knee bent: WNL

**Knee**

Right knee flexion: pain at end range

Right knee extension: pain at end range

Right knee tibial internal rotation: 20 degrees (left is 40 degrees)

**Ankle**

Right ankle dorsiflexion: −10 degrees (left is +5 degrees)

**Joint play**

Empty

**Special tests**

Thomas + right; McMurray's + right

**Manual muscle testing**

Core: WNL

Psoas: 3/5 right with pain

Popliteus: 3/5 right with pain

**Neurodynamic assessment**

WNL

**Tight tender points/soft tissue restrictions**

Right: psoas; iliacus; gastroc—trigger points

Right: psoas; iliacus; sartorius; popliteus; gastroc—soft tissue restrictions

**Posture**

WNL

**Ergonomics**

WNL

## ASSESSMENT

The patient presents with signs and symptoms consistent with a meniscus tear. The patient presents with an increase in symptoms with walking, climbing stairs, prolonged sit to stand, and stiffness first thing in the morning. Trigger points in right psoas; iliacus, and gastroc. Soft tissue restrictions noted in right sartorius, gastroc, psoas, and iliacus. Popliteus weakness was noted along with weakness in psoas with pain. Decreased range of motion in right tibial internal rotation, ankle dorsiflexion, and hip extension.

### Plan

Self–myofascial release/corrective flexibility/corrective exercises/corrective manual therapy/modalities

---

### Self–Myofascial Release

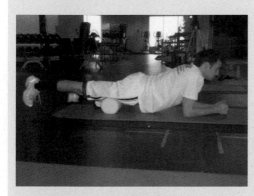

**FIGURE 26.1A.** Foam roll: right rectus femoris, gastroc.

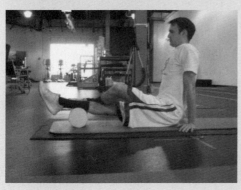

**FIGURE 26.1B.** Foam roll: right gastroc.

*(continued)*

## Self–Myofascial Release (*continued*)

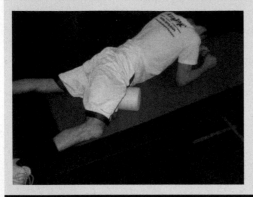

**FIGURE 26.1C.** Foam roll: right adductors.

## Corrective Flexibility

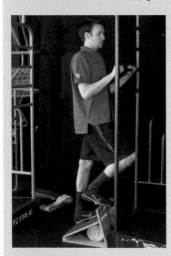

**FIGURE 26.2A.** Static: right gastroc.

(*continued*)

# Corrective Flexibility (*continued*)

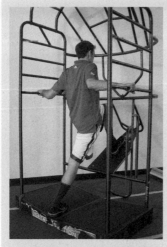

**FIGURE 26.2B.** Static: right hip flexors.

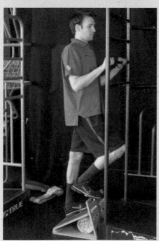

**FIGURE 26.2C.** Active: bilateral iastroc.

(*continued*)

## Corrective Flexibility (*continued*)

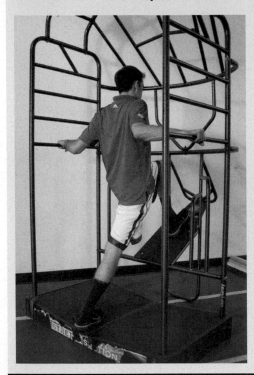

**FIGURE 26.2D.** Active: bilateral hip flexors.

## Corrective Exercise

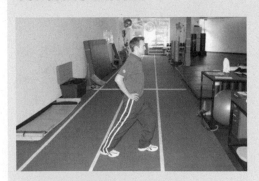

**FIGURE 26.3A.** Split stance: anterior knee drive.

(*continued*)

## Corrective Exercise (*continued*)

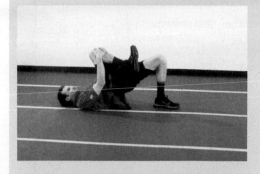

**FIGURE 26.3B.** Bridge: leg lock bridge (right 2:1).

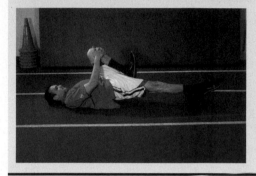

**FIGURE 26.3C.** Bridge: leg lock with knee straight on foam roll (right 2:1).

## Manual Therapy

1. Warming technique: gastroc, popliteus
2. Inhibitory technique: right, psoas, and iliacus
3. Elongation technique: right psoas and iliacus; gastroc; popliteus

## Modalities

1. Ice prn

## Home Exercise Program

1. Foam roll: right rectus femoris and gastroc
2. Ice: prn

Orthopedic and Rehabilitation Associates
Orthopedic Street
Omaha, OH
(555) 555-5555
Fax. (666) 666-7777

PATIENT: *Mr. O*
DATE: *2009*

## ORTHOPAEDIC REHABILITATION PRESCRIPTION

*REHAB THERAPIES*   ☒ PT   ☐ OT   ☐ SESSIONS/WK *2*
TOTAL *12*

☒ NEW DIAGNOSIS   ☐ RE-EVALUATION   ☒ OUTPATIENT

DIAGNOSIS1 *Meniscus tear*
    ICD _____

DIAGNOSIS2 _____
    ICD _____

PREGNANT? ☐ YES ☒ NO        PERTINENTMEDICALHISTORY: *None*

GOALS:
MD/DO: ☒ INCREASE MOBILITY ☒ INCREASE ADL ☒ INCREASE STRENGTH ☒ DECREASE PAIN

PRECAUTIONS: ☐ CARDIAC    MAX-SBP_____ DBP_____ HR_____
ABOVE BASELINE    ☐ DIABETES: HYPER/HYPOGLYCEMIA ☐ ORTHOSTASIS
☐ OTHER _____

WEIGHT BEARING:   ☐ WBAT   ☐ TTWB   ☐ NWB
    TO: _____

MODALITIES: ☐ ULTRASOUND TO: *RLE x 7 min*
              ☐ E-STIM    TO: *RLE x 7 min B/L*

        ☐ FLUID THERAPY    ☐ JOBST      ☐ PARAFFIN
    TO: _____
        ☐ ICE    TO: *10 min to R knee*

        ☐ HOTPACKS    TO: *10 min to R knee*
        ☐ EXERCISES ☐ PROM ☐ AAROM ☐ AROM
    TO: *B/L LE*
        ☒ PRE's   ☐ ISOMETRICS   ☐ ISOKINETICS
    TO: *BL L/E*
        ☐ SLIDEBOARD ☐ PLYOMETRICS ☐ MODIFIED KNEE BEND
☐ STEPUPS
☒ LUMBAR STABILIZATION ☐ WILLIAM's ☐ McKENZIE ☐ CERVICAL EXERCISES
☐ RELAXATION ☐ COORDINATION
MANUAL: ☒ CONTRACT RELAX ☐ CRANIOSACRAL ☒ JONES/C-STRAIN ☒ SOFT
TISSUE MOBILIZATION
        ☒ STRETCHING ☒ MASSAGE ☒ MYOF AS RELEASE ☒ SPRAY/STRETCH
    TO: *LE B/L Cervicalparaspinals*
EDUCATION: ☒ MOBILITY: ☐ TRANSFERS ☒ ADL ☒ HEP ☐ ENERGY CONSERV
☐ WORK HARDENING ☒ BIOMECHANICS ☐ 1
HANDED TECHNIQUES
☐ GAIT TRAINING ☐ FINE MOTOR ☐ COORD/BALANCE
OTHER: _____

_____
_____

ADL-ACTIVITIES OF DAILY LIVING     AAROM-ACTIVE/ASSISTIVERANGEOFMOTION   DBP-
DIASTOLIC BLOOD PRESSURE
SBP-SYSTOLIC BLOOD PRESSURE    HR-HEART RATE    HEP-HOME EXERCISE PROGRAM
NWB-NON-WEIGHT BEARING
PRE's-PROGRESSIVE RESISTIVE EXERCISES    WBAT-WEIGHT BEARING AS TOLERATED
ROM-RANGE OF MOTION

The above is medically necessary to decrease debility and achieve ADL independence. Also to:
☒ decrease pain, ☒ improve strength/endurance, ☒ improve balance coordination, ☒ improve gait,
☒ improve transfers,
Other _____

PHYSICIAN'S SIGNATURE _____ DATE _____

# CASE **27**

## PATELLOFEMORAL SYNDROME

**CC:** Knee pain

**HPI:** Ms. R is 28 years old and an avid runner. She has been training for the New York City marathon and increasing her mileage slowly. Her right knee began hurting 6 weeks ago. The more she ignores it, the more it hurts. The knee is now painful when running, or even walking for prolonged periods of time. If sitting for more than 15 minutes, her knee becomes achy and she needs to straighten it. The pain is primarily in the front of the knee. She has not taken any pain medications or had any x-rays. No locking, catching, or giving way of the knees.

**PMHx:** None

**PSHx:** None

**Meds:** None

**Allergies:** PCN but she is not sure what happens when she takes it.

**Social:** No tobacco. Social EtOH

**ROS:** Noncontributory

## PHYSICAL EXAMINATION

On exam, Ms. R is a well-developed female who looks her stated age. BP: 110/64, P: 58, RR: 14. She has 5/5 strength, intact sensation, and 2+ patella and Achilles reflexes in the bilateral lower extremities. No swelling or ecchymosis is present. No joint line tenderness bilaterally. Peripatellar tenderness of the right knee is noted. Positive J-sign bilaterally. No crepitus. No instability is noted. McMurray and Apley compression and distraction tests are negative. The left knee exam is within normal limits. 2+ distal pulses are palpated bilaterally.

### Impression

Right patellofemoral syndrome.

### Plan

1. Physical therapy

# PHYSICAL THERAPY

The patient is a 28-year-old female who injured her right knee × 6 weeks ago while training for the New York City marathon. The patient went to the medical doctor who referred her to physical therapy. Pain is in the right inferior lateral patella.

**Scale:** 2/10 pain at rest; 6–7/10 with running
**Increase pain:** running; climbing stairs; squatting
**Decrease pain:** sitting; rest

## Range of Motion

**Hip**
Left hip extension: WNL
Right hip extension: –10 degrees
Left hip flexion with knee bent: WNL
Right hip flexion with knee bent: WNL
Right hip IR: 15 degrees (left 30 degrees)
**Knee**
Right knee flexion: WNL
Right knee extension: WNL
**Ankle**
Right ankle dorsiflexion: WNL
**Joint play**
WNL
**Special tests**
Thomas + right; Ober's + right
**Manual muscle testing**
Core: WNL
Psoas: 3/5 right
Tensor fascia latae: 3/5 right with pain
**Neurodynamic assessment**
WNL
**Tight tender points/soft tissue restrictions**
Right: psoas; iliacus; vastus lateralis—trigger points
Right: psoas; iliacus; vastus lateralis; iliotibial band—soft tissue restrictions
**Posture**
WNL
**Ergonomics**
WNL

## ASSESSMENT

The patient presents with signs and symptoms consistent with patella-femoral syndrome. The patient presents with an increase in symptoms with running, climbing stairs, and squatting. Trigger points in right psoas; iliacus, and vastus lateralis. Soft tissue restrictions noted in right vastus lateralis and iliotibial band, psoas, and iliacus. Tensor fascia latae weakness was noted along with weakness in psoas. Decreased range of motion in right femoral internal rotation and hip extension noted.

### Plan

Self–myofascial release/corrective flexibility/corrective exercises/corrective manual therapy/modalities

### Self–Myofascial Release

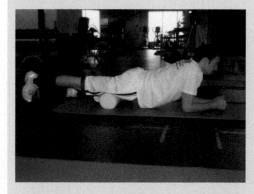

**FIGURE 27.1A.** Foam roll: right rectus femoris.

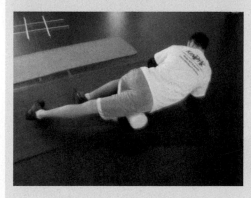

**FIGURE 27.1B.** Foam roll: right vastus lateralis.

(*continued*)

## Self–Myofascial Release (*continued*)

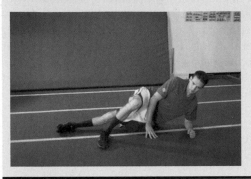

**FIGURE 27.1C.** Foam roll: right iliotibial band.

## Corrective Flexibility

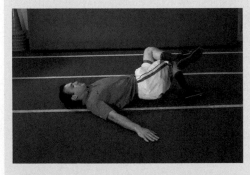

**FIGURE 27.2A.** Static: right iliotibial band in hooklying.

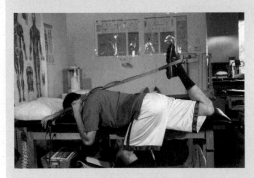

**FIGURE 27.2B.** Static: right rectus femoris.

(*continued*)

# Corrective Flexibility (*continued*)

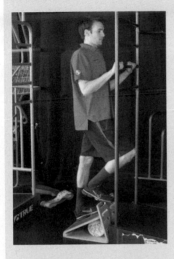

**FIGURE 27.2C.** Active: bilateral gastroc.

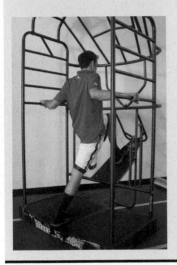

**FIGURE 27.2D.** Active: bilateral hip flexors.

## Corrective Exercise

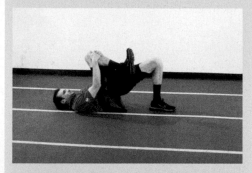

**FIGURE 27.3A.** Bridge: leg lock bridge (right 2:1).

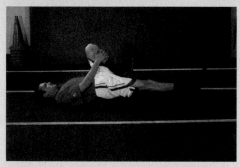

**FIGURE 27.3B.** Bridge: leg lock with knee straight on foam roll (right 2:1).

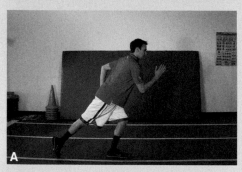

**FIGURE 27.3(A-B).** Single leg runner's technique.

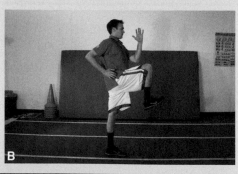

## ManualTherapy

1. Warming technique: right rectus femoris, iliotibial band
2. Inhibitory technique: right psoas and iliacus
3. Activation technique: right vastus lateralis
4. Elongation technique: right psoas and iliacus; vastus lateralis and iliotibial band

## Modalities

None

## Home Exercise Program

1. Tennis ball: right rectus femoris, iliotibial band
2. Static: right iliotibial band

PATIENT: _Ms. R_
DATE: _2009_

# ORTHOPAEDIC REHABILITATION PRESCRIPTION

**_REHAB THERAPIES_**  ☒ PT  ☐ OT  ☐ SESSIONS/WK _2_
TOTAL _12_

☐ NEW DIAGNOSIS  ☒ RE-EVALUATION  ☒ OUTPATIENT

DIAGNOSIS1 _Left quadriceps strain_
　ICD _____

DIAGNOSIS2 _____
　ICD _____

PREGNANT? ☐ YES ☒ NO　　PERTINENT MEDICAL HISTORY: _____

GOALS:
MD/DO: ☒ INCREASE MOBILITY ☒ INCREASE ADL ☒ INCREASE STRENGTH ☒ DECREASE PAIN

PRECAUTIONS: ☐ CARDIAC　MAX-SBP _____ DBP _____ HR _____
ABOVE BASELINE　☐ DIABETES: HYPER/HYPOGLYCEMIA ☐ ORTHOSTASIS
☐ OTHER _____
WEIGHT BEARING:　☐ WBAT　☐ TTWB　☐ NWB
　TO: _____
MODALITIES: ☐ ULTRASOUND TO: _Left thigh x 7 min_
　　　　　☐ E-STIM　TO: _Left thigh hand x 7 min B/L_
B/L _____
　　☐ FLUID THERAPY　☐ JOBST　☐ PARAFFIN
　TO: _____
　　☐ ICE　TO: _10 min to L thigh_
B/L _____
　　☐ HOTPACKS　TO: _10 min to L thigh_
　　☐ EXERCISES ☐ PROM ☐ AAROM ☐ AROM
　TO: _____
　　☐ PRE's ☐ ISOMETRICS ☐ ISOKINETICS
　TO: _B/L LE_
　　☐ SLIDEBOARD ☐ PLYOMETRICS ☐ MODIFIED KNEE BEND
☐ STEPUPS
☒ LUMBAR STABILIZATION ☐ WILLIAM's ☐ McKENZIE ☐ CERVICAL EXERCISES
☐ RELAXATION ☐ COORDINATION
MANUAL: ☒ CONTRACT RELAX ☐ CRANIOSACRAL ☒ JONES/C-STRAIN ☒ SOFT
TISSUE MOBILIZATION
　　☒ STRETCHING ☒ MASSAGE ☒ MYOFAS RELEASE ☒ SPRAY/STRETCH
　TO: _LE B/L_
EDUCATION: ☒ MOBILITY: ☐ TRANSFERS ☒ ADL ☒ HEP ☐ ENERGY CONSERV
☐ WORK HARDENING ☒ BIOMECHANICS ☐ 1 HANDED TECHNIQUES
☐ GAIT TRAINING ☐ FINE MOTOR ☐ COORD/BALANCE
OTHER: _____

The above is medically necessary to decrease debility and achieve ADL independence. Also to:
☒ decrease pain, ☒ improve strength/endurance, ☒ improve balance coordination, ☒ improve gait,
☒ improve transfers,
Other _____
PHYSICIAN'S SIGNATURE _____ DATE _____

# CASE 28

# KNEE OSTEOARTHRITIS

**CC:** Knee pain

**HPI:** Mr. T is 62 years old and complains of a 6 week history of dull, aching left knee pain. The pain is worse with stair climbing and better with lying flat. When sitting for a prolonged period of time, the knee bothers him until he straightens it. Long distance walking also makes the pain worse. He takes an occasional Tylenol for the pain, which helps a little. On average, the pain is 4/10 intensity. He has not had any imaging studies of his knees. No locking, catching, or giving way of the knees.

**PMHx:** HTN

**PSHx:** None

**Meds:** HCTZ

**Allergies:** NKDA

**Social:** No tobacco. Social EtOH

**ROS:** Noncontributory

## PHYSICAL EXAMINATION

On exam, Mr. T is a muscular male who looks his stated age. BP: 128/82, P: 64, RR: 14. He has 5/5 strength, intact sensation, and 2+ patella and Achilles reflexes in the bilateral lower extremities. No swelling or ecchymosis is present. No joint line or peripatellar tenderness bilaterally. Negative J-sign bilaterally. Positive crepitus in the knees, left more than right. No instability is noted. McMurray and Apley compression and distraction tests are negative. 2+ distal pulses are palpated bilaterally.

## Impression

Right knee osteoarthritis

## Plan

1. X-ray B/L knees
2. Physical therapy

# PHYSICAL THERAPY

The patient is a 62-year-old male who complains of right knee pain that started 6 weeks ago. The patient says it is an insidious onset. The patient went to the physician who referred the patient to physical therapy to treat for knee osteoarthritis.

**Scale:** 4/10 pain at rest
**Increase pain:** climbing stairs; squatting; prolonged sitting and walking
**Decrease pain:** sitting; rest with knee straight

## Range of Motion

**Hip**
Left hip extension: WNL
Right hip extension: −10 degrees
Left hip flexion with knee bent: WNL
Right hip flexion with knee bent: WNL
Right hip IR: 0 degree (left 25 degrees)
**Knee**
Right knee flexion: 115 degrees with pain
Right knee extension: WNL
**Ankle**
Right ankle dorsiflexion: WNL
**Joint play**
Right anterior knee glide is 2/6
**Special tests**
Thomas + right
**Manual muscle testing**
Core: WNL
Psoas: 3/5 right
Medial hamstring: 3/5 right with pain
**Neurodynamic assessment**
WNL
**Tight tender points/soft tissue restrictions**
Right: psoas; iliacus; vastus lateralis rectus femoris—trigger points
Right: psoas; iliacus; vastus lateralis; medial hamstring—soft tissue restrictions
**Posture**
WNL
**Ergonomics**
WNL

## ASSESSMENT

The patient presents with signs and symptoms consistent with right knee osteoarthritis. The patient presents with an increase in symptoms with prolonged sitting and walking, climbing stairs, and squatting. Trigger points in right psoas; iliacus, rectus femoris, and vastus lateralis. Soft tissue restrictions noted in right vastus lateralis, medial hamstring, psoas, and iliacus. Medial hamstring weakness was noted along with weakness in psoas. Decreased range of motion in right femoral internal rotation and hip extension noted.

### Plan

Self–myofascial release/corrective flexibility/corrective exercises/corrective manual therapy/modalities

---

### Self–Myofascial Release

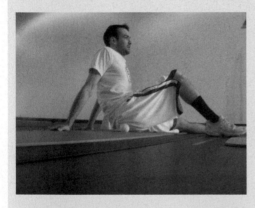

**FIGURE 28.1A.** Tennis ball: right piriformis.

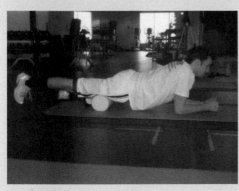

**FIGURE 28.1B.** Foam roll: right rectus femoris.

*(continued)*

## Self–Myofascial Release (*continued*)

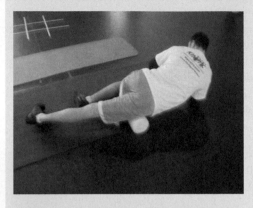

**FIGURE 28.1C.** Foam roll: right vastus lateralis.

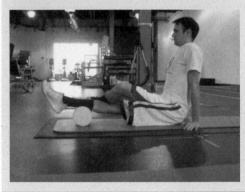

**FIGURE 28.1D.** Foam roll: right gastroc.

## Corrective Flexibility

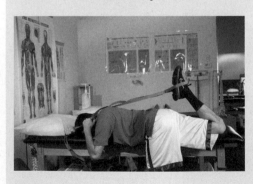

**FIGURE 28.2A.** Static: right rectus femoris prone on table.

(*continued*)

## Corrective Flexibility (*continued*)

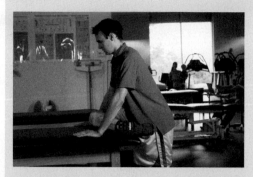

**FIGURE 28.2B.** Static: right piriformis leg on table.

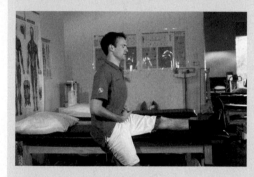

**FIGURE 28.2C.** Static medial hamstring on table in sitting position.

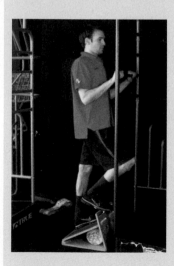

**FIGURE 28.2D.** Active: bilateral gastroc.

(*continued*)

## Corrective Flexibility (*continued*)

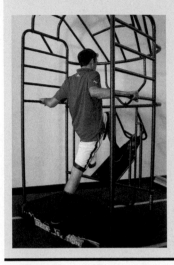

**FIGURE 28.2E.** Active: bilateral hip flexors.

## Corrective Exercise

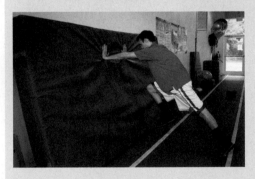

**FIGURE 28.3A.** Wall push: knee to chest.

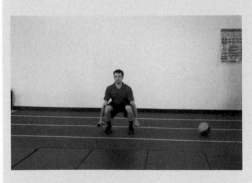

**FIGURE 28.3B.** Squat technique.

(*continued*)

## Corrective Exercise (*continued*)

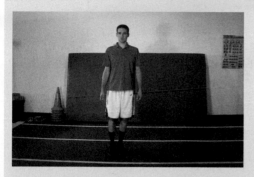

**FIGURE 28.3C.** Single balance reach: 3D.

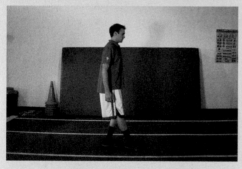

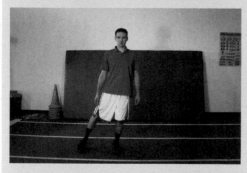

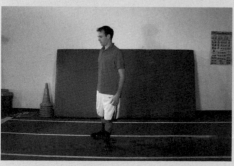

## Manual Therapy

1. Warming technique: right rectus femoris, iliotibial band, vastus lateralis
2. Inhibitory technique: right psoas and iliacus
3. Activation technique: right vastus lateralis, vastus medialis oblique
4. Elongation technique: right psoas and iliacus, vastus lateralis, iliotibial band, medial hamstring
5. Hip mobilizations to improve internal rotation
6. Anterior tibial mobilizations to improve knee flexion

## Modalities

1. Heat prn

## Home Exercise Program

1. Tennis ball: right rectus femoris, iliotibial band, gastroc
2. Static: right rectus femoris prone on bed
3. Heat prn

Orthopedic and Rehabilitation Associates
Orthopedic Street
Omaha, OH
(555) 555-5555
Fax. (666) 666-7777

PATIENT: _Mr. T_
DATE: _2009_

## ORTHOPAEDIC REHABILITATION PRESCRIPTION

| REHAB THERAPIES | ☒ PT | ☐ OT | ☐ SESSIONS/WK _2_ |
| --- | --- | --- | --- |

TOTAL _12_

☒ NEW DIAGNOSIS    ☐ RE-EVALUATION    ☒ OUTPATIENT

DIAGNOSIS1 _Knee Osteoarthritis_
  ICD _____

DIAGNOSIS2 _____
  ICD _____

PREGNANT? ☐ YES ☒ NO        PERTINENT MEDICAL HISTORY: _HTN_

GOALS:
MD/DO: ☒ INCREASE MOBILITY ☒ INCREASE ADL ☒ INCREASE STRENGTH ☒ DECREASE PAIN

PRECAUTIONS: ☐ CARDIAC    MAX-SBP _20_ DBP _10_ HR _20_
ABOVE BASELINE    ☐ DIABETES: HYPER/HYPOGLYCEMIA ☐ ORTHOSTASIS
☐ OTHER _____
WEIGHT BEARING: ☐ WBAT ☐ TTWB ☐ NWB
  TO: _____
MODALITIES: ☐ ULTRASOUND TO: _LLE x 7 min_
            ☐ E-STIM        TO: _LLE x 7 min B/L_

            ☐ FLUID THERAPY    ☐ JOBST    ☐ PARAFFIN
  TO: _____
            ☐ ICE    TO: _10 min to L knee_

            ☐ HOTPACKS    TO: _10 min to L knee_
            ☐ EXERCISES ☐ PROM ☐ AAROM ☐ AROM
  TO: _B L/E_
            ☒ PRE's ☐ ISOMETRICS ☐ ISOKINETICS
  TO: _B L/E_
            ☐ SLIDEBOARD ☐ PLYOMETRICS ☐ MODIFIED KNEE BEND
☐ STEPUPS
☒ LUMBAR STABILIZATION ☐ WILLIAM's ☐ McKENZIE ☐ CERVICAL EXERCISES
☐ RELAXATION ☐ COORDINATION
MANUAL: ☒ CONTRACT RELAX ☐ CRANIOSACRAL ☒ JONES/C-STRAIN ☒ SOFT
TISSUE MOBILIZATION
            ☒ STRETCHING ☒ MASSAGE ☒ MYOF AS RELEASE ☒ SPRAY/STRETCH
  TO: _LE B/L_
EDUCATION: ☒ MOBILITY: ☐ TRANSFERS ☒ ADL ☒ HEP ☐ ENERGY CONSERV
☐ WORK HARDENING ☒ BIOMECHANICS ☐ 1
HANDED TECHNIQUES
☐ GAIT TRAINING ☐ FINE MOTOR ☐ COORD/BALANCE
OTHER: _____
_____
_____

ADL-ACTIVITIES OF DAILY LIVING    AAROM-ACTIVE/ASSISTIVE RANGE OF MOTION   DBP-
DIASTOLIC BLOOD PRESSURE
SBP-SYSTOLIC BLOOD PRESSURE   HR-HEART RATE   HEP-HOME EXERCISE PROGRAM
NWB-NON-WEIGHT BEARING
PRE's-PROGRESSIVE RESISTIVE EXERCISES   WBAT-WEIGHT BEARING AS TOLERATED
ROM-RANGE OF MOTION

The above is medically necessary to decrease debility and achieve ADL independence. Also to:
☒ decrease pain, ☒ improve strength/endurance, ☒ improve balance coordination, ☒ improve gait,
☒ improve transfers,
Other _____

PHYSICIAN'S SIGNATURE _____ DATE _____

# CASE 29

# DEGENERATIVE MENISCUS TEAR

**CC:** Left knee pain

**HPI:** Mr. E is 66 years old and complains of 4 months of left knee pain. He has always had an "aching" in the knees, but 4 months ago the left knee got worse. No inciting event. Two months ago, the left knee "locked" and it took about 5 minutes of massaging it for the knee to unlock. Since then, no locking incidents. No giving way of the knee. Sitting is more painful. Climbing stairs is also painful. The pain is 3/10 while sitting and 6–7/10 while going down stairs. Rest makes the pain better. He has not noted any bruising or swelling of the knee.

**PMHx:** High cholesterol

**PSHx:** None

**Meds:** Niacin

**Allergies:** NKDA

**Social:** No tobacco. Social EtOH

**ROS:** Noncontributory

## PHYSICAL EXAMINATION

On exam, Mr. E is an overweight male who looks his stated age. BP: 136/88, P: 70, RR: 14. He has 5/5 strength, intact sensation, and 2+ patella and Achilles reflexes in the bilateral lower extremities. A small effusion is noted over the left knee. No ecchymosis is present. Medial joint line tenderness is noted over the left knee. No peripatellar tenderness is noted. Negative

J-sign bilaterally. Positive crepitus in the knees bilaterally. No instability is noted bilaterally. McMurray and Apley compression tests are positive on the left but not on the right. 2+ distal pulses are palpated bilaterally.

## Impression

Degenerative meniscus tear

**Plan**

1. MRI left knee
2. Physical therapy

# PHYSICAL THERAPY

The patient is 66 years old who presents with left knee pain that started 4 months ago. Pain has gotten progressively worse with an insidious onset. The patient went to the physician who referred the patient to physical therapy. The patient currently reports that feeling of locking in his left knee.

**Scale:** 3/10 pain at rest; 6–7/10 while descending stairs
**Increase pain:** climbing/descending stairs; squatting; prolonged sitting
**Decrease pain:** sitting;

## Range of Motion

**Hip**
WNL
**Knee**
Left knee flexion: 125 degrees with pain
Left knee extension: WNL
**Ankle**
Right ankle dorsiflexion: WNL
**Joint play**
Empty
**Special tests**
Apley compression: + left
**Manual muscle testing**
Core: WNL
Psoas: WNL
Medial hamstring: 3/5 left with pain
Popliteus: 3/5 left with pain
**Neurodynamic assessment**
WNL
**Tight tender points/soft tissue restrictions**
Left: popliteus; sartorius; adductor longus—trigger points
Left: medial hamstring; popliteus—soft tissue restrictions
**Posture**
WNL
**Ergonomics**
WNL

## ASSESSMENT

The patient presents with signs and symptoms consistent with left knee medial meniscus tear. The patient presents with an increase in symptoms with squatting; ascending/descending stairs, and prolonged sitting. Trigger points in left popliteus, sartorius, and adductor longus. Soft tissue restrictions noted in left medial hamstring and popliteus. Medial hamstring and popliteus weakness was noted. Decreased range of motion in left knee flexion noted with pain.

### Plan

Self–myofascial release/corrective flexibility/corrective exercises/corrective manual therapy/modalities

### Self–Myofascial Release

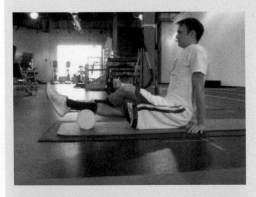

**FIGURE 29.1A.** Foam roll: left medial gastroc.

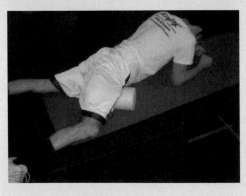

**FIGURE 29.1B.** Foam roll: left adductors and medial hamstrings.

*(continued)*

## Self Myofascial Release (*continued*)

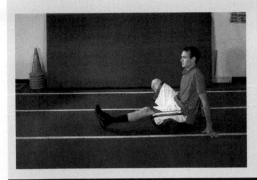

**FIGURE 29.1C.** Foam roll: left medial hamstring.

## Corrective Flexibility

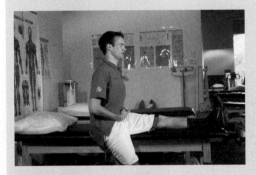

**FIGURE 29.2A.** Static: left medial hamstring on table.

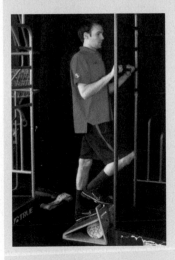

**FIGURE 29.2B.** Static: left gastroc.

(*continued*)

# Corrective Flexibility (*continued*)

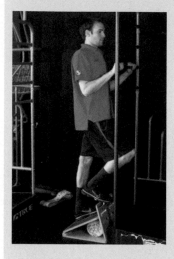

**FIGURE 29.2C.** Active: bilateral gastroc.

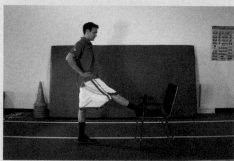

**FIGURE 29.2D.** Active: bilateral hamstrings 3D on chair.

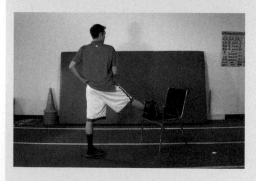

(*continued*)

## Corrective Flexibility (*continued*)

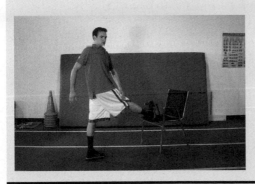

## Corrective Exercise

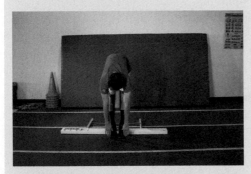

**FIGURE 29.3A.** Progressive hamstring.

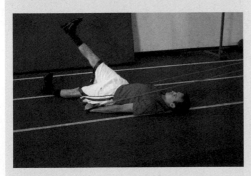

**FIGURE 29.3B.** SLR with core activation.

(*continued*)

## Corrective Exercise (*continued*)

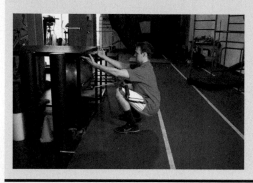

**FIGURE 29.3C.** Squat with adduction.

### Manual Therapy

1. Warming technique: left medial hamstring. Adductors, medial gastroc
2. Inhibitory technique: left popliteus
3. Activation technique: left medial hamstring at distal attachment
4. Elongation technique: left medial hamstring, sartorius, and popliteus

### Modalities: prn

### Home Exercise Program

1. Tennis ball: left medial gastroc
2. Foam roll: left adductors
3. Static: left medial hamstring on bed

Orthopedic and Rehabilitation Associates
Orthopedic Street
Omaha, OH
(555) 555-5555
Fax. (666) 666-7777

PATIENT: *Mr. E*
DATE: *2009*

## ORTHOPAEDIC REHABILITATION PRESCRIPTION

**REHAB THERAPIES**   ☒ PT   ☐ OT   ☐ SESSIONS/WK _*2*_
TOTAL *12*

☒ NEW DIAGNOSIS   ☐ RE-EVALUATION   ☒ OUTPATIENT

DIAGNOSIS1 _*Degenerative Meniscus Tear*_
  ICD _____

DIAGNOSIS2 _____
  ICD _____

PREGNANT? ☐ YES ☒ NO      PERTINENTMEDICALHISTORY: *None*

GOALS:
MD/DO: ☒ INCREASE MOBILITY ☒ INCREASE ADL ☒ INCREASE STRENGTH ☒ DECREASE PAIN

PRECAUTIONS: ☐ CARDIAC   MAX-SBP ____ DBP ____ HR ____
ABOVE BASELINE   ☐ DIABETES: HYPER/HYPOGLYCEMIA ☐ ORTHOSTASIS
☐ OTHER _____

WEIGHT BEARING: ☐ WBAT ☐ TTWB ☐ NWB
  TO: _____

MODALITIES: ☐ ULTRASOUND TO: *LLE x 7 min*
    ☐ E-STIM   TO: *LLE x 7 min B/L*

  ☐ FLUID THERAPY   ☐ JOBST   ☐ PARAFFIN
  TO: _____
    ☐ ICE   TO: *10 min to L knee*

    ☐ HOTPACKS   TO: *10 min to L knee*
    ☐ EXERCISES ☐ PROM ☐ AAROM ☐ AROM
  TO: *B/L LE*
    ☒ PRE's ☐ SOMETRICS ☐ SOKINETICS
  TO: *B/L LE*
    ☐ SLIDEBOARD ☐ PLYOMETRICS ☐ MODIFIED KNEE BEND
☐ STEPUPS
☒ LUMBAR STABILIZATION ☐ WILLIAM's ☐ McKENZIE ☐ CERVICAL EXERCISES
☐ RELAXATION ☐ COORDINATION
MANUAL: ☒ CONTRACT RELAX ☐ CRANIOSACRAL ☒ JONES/C-STRAIN ☒ SOFT
TISSUE MOBILIZATION
    ☒ STRETCHING ☒ MASSAGE ☒ MYOF AS RELEASE ☒ SPRAY/STRETCH
  TO: *LE B/L*
    ☐ SLIDEBOARD
EDUCATION: ☒ MOBILITY: ☐ TRANSFERS ☒ ADL ☒ HEP ☐ ENERGY CONSERV
  ☐ WORK HARDENING ☒ BIOMECHANICS ☐ 1
HANDED TECHNIQUES
  ☐ GAIT TRAINING ☐ FINE MOTOR ☐ COORD/BALANCE
OTHER: _____
_____
_____

ADL-ACTIVITIES OF DAILY LIVING   AAROM-ACTIVE/ASSISTIVERANGEOFMOTION   DBP-
DIASTOLIC BLOOD PRESSURE
SBP-SYSTOLIC BLOOD PRESSURE   HR-HEART RATE   HEP-HOME EXERCISE PROGRAM
NWB-NON-WEIGHT BEARING
PRE's-PROGRESSIVE RESISTIVE EXERCISES   WBAT-WEIGHT BEARING AS TOLERATED
ROM-RANGE OF MOTION

The above is medically necessary to decrease debility and achieve ADL independence. Also to:
☒ decrease pain, ☒ improve strength/endurance, ☒ improve balance coordination, ☒ improve gait,
☒ improve transfers,
Other _____

PHYSICIAN'S SIGNATURE _____ DATE _____

# PART 9

## LOWER LEG PAIN

# CASE 30

# COMPARTMENT SYNDROME

**CC:** Left anterior-lateral calf pain

**HPI:** Mr. F is a 32-year-old amateur marathon runner. He had been training for the Philadelphia marathon and noticed that after 10 miles, he would develop a severe pain in his left anterior-lateral calf. The pain would get worse until he rested. As soon as he stopped running, the pain would subside. If he tried running again, the pain would quickly return. He kept training, but in the last week, the pain started after only 2 miles. The marathon is in 1 month and he is concerned that he will not be able to participate. He denies any numbness, tingling, or burning. No weakness. He has never had a problem like this before and he has been running since high school.

**PMHx:** None
**PSHx:** None
**Meds:** None
**Allergies:** NKDA
**Social:** No tobacco. Social EtOH
**ROS:** Noncontributory

## PHYSICAL EXAMINATION

On exam, Mr. F is a well-developed, fit male who looks his stated age. BP: 114/74, P: 60, RR: 14. He has 5/5 strength, intact sensation, and 2+ patella and Achilles reflexes in the bilateral lower extremities. 2+ distal pulses are palpated bilaterally. There is no swelling or ecchymosis in his lower extremities bilaterally. No tenderness over his calves. No bony tenderness.

## Impression

Chronic compartment syndrome

## Plan

1. Schedule compartment pressure test
2. Physical therapy

# PHYSICAL THERAPY

The patient is a 32-year-old male runner who presents with left anterior-lateral calf pain that started a week ago. The patient noticed while training for a marathon that after the 10th mile he started to feel severe pain. The patient was referred to physical therapy with a diagnosis of chronic compartment syndrome.

Scale: 10/10 pain

**Increase pain:** running >2 miles

**Decrease pain:** not running

## Range of Motion

**Hip**

Hip extension: left 10 degrees

Hip extension: right 0 degree

**Knee**

Left knee flexion: WNL

Left knee extension: WNL

**Ankle**

Right ankle dorsiflexion: WNL

Left ankle dorsiflexion: –5 degrees

**Manual muscle testing**

WNL

**Neurodynamic assessment**

WNL

**Tight tender points/soft tissue restrictions**

Left: gastroc, anterior tibialis, vastus lateralis—trigger points

Left: anterior tibialis, biceps femoris, vastus lateralis—soft tissue restrictions

**Posture**

WNL

**Ergonomics**

WNL

## ASSESSMENT

The patient presents with signs and symptoms consistent with left compartment syndrome. The patient presents with an increase in symptoms with running. Trigger points in left gastroc, anterior tibialis, and vastus lateralis. Soft tissue restrictions noted in left anterior tibialis, biceps femoris, and vastus lateralis.

### Plan

Self–myofascial release/corrective flexibility/corrective exercises/corrective manual therapy/modalities

## Self–Myofascial Release

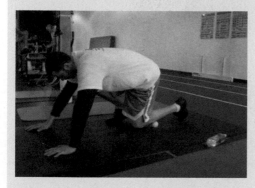

**FIGURE 30.1A.** Tennis ball: left anterior tibialis.

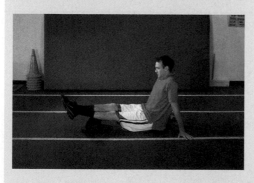

**FIGURE 30.1B.** Foam roll: peroneus longus.

(*continued*)

## Self–Myofascial Release (*continued*)

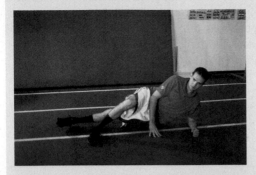

**FIGURE 30.1C.** Foam roll: iliotibial band.

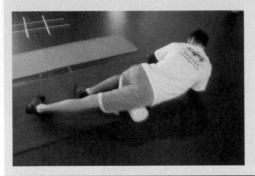

**FIGURE 30.1D.** Foam roll: vastus lateralis.

## Corrective Flexibility

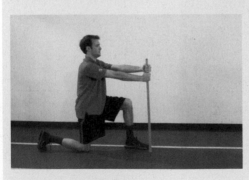

**FIGURE 30.2A.** Static: left rectus femoris in kneeling.

(*continued*)

## Corrective Flexibility (*continued*)

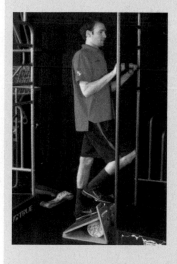

**FIGURE 30.2B.** Static: left gastroc.

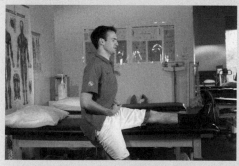

**FIGURE 30.2C.** Static: left lateral hamstring in sitting.

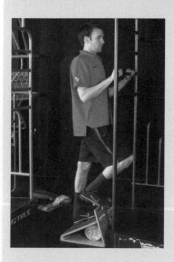

**FIGURE 30.2D.** Active: bilateral gastroc.

(*continued*)

## Corrective Flexibility (*continued*)

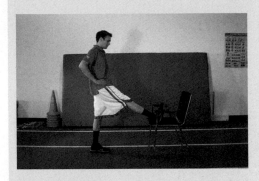

**FIGURE 30.2E.** Active: bilateral hamstrings 3D on chair.

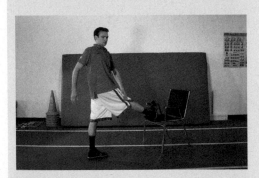

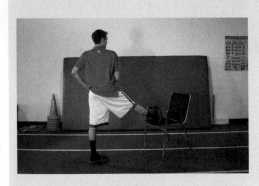

*(continued)*

## Corrective Flexibility (*continued*)

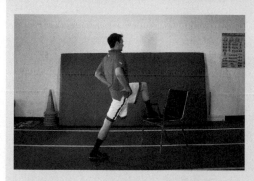

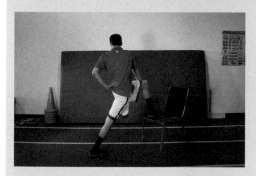

**FIGURE 30.2F.** Active: bilateral hip flexor 3D on chair.

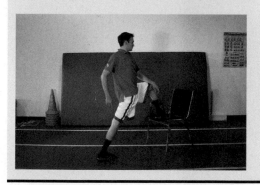

## Corrective Exercise

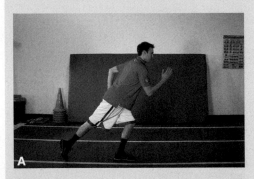

**FIGURE 30.3(A–B).** Running techniques on single leg.

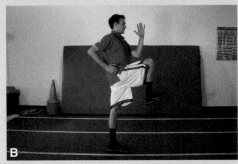

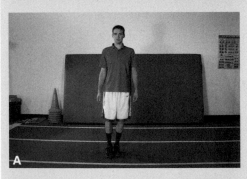

**FIGURE 30.4(A–D).** Balance reach: BD.

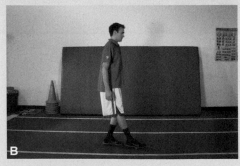

(*continued*)

## Corrective Exercise (*continued*)

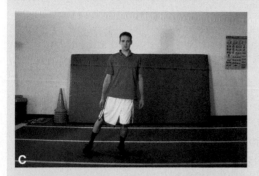

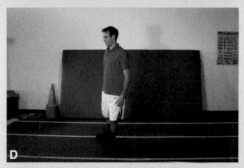

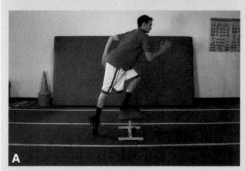

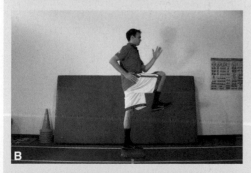

**FIGURE 30.5(A–B).** Step up technique.

## Manual Therapy

1. Warming technique: left vastus lateralis, iliotibial band, biceps femoris, anterior tibialis
2. Inhibitory technique: left anterior tibialis
3. Activation technique: left anterior tibialis proximal attachment
4. Elongation technique: left vastus lateralis, biceps femoris, anterior tibialis

## Modalities

## Home Exercise Program

1. Tennis ball: left anterior tibialis, vastus lateralis, iliotibial band
2. Static: left bicep femoris in sitting on table
3. Static: left iliotibial band in hooklying

Orthopedic and Rehabilitation Associates
Orthopedic Street
Omaha, OH
(555) 555-5555
Fax. (666) 666-7777

PATIENT: *Mr. F*
DATE: *2009*

## ORTHOPAEDIC REHABILITATION PRESCRIPTION

*REHAB THERAPIES*  ☒ PT  ☐ OT  ☐ SESSIONS/WK *2*
TOTAL *12*

☒ NEW DIAGNOSIS  ☐ RE-EVALUATION  ☒ OUTPATIENT

DIAGNOSIS1 *Chronic Compartment Syndrome*
ICD _____

DIAGNOSIS2 _____
ICD _____

PREGNANT?  ☐ YES  ☒ NO  PERTINENTMEDICALHISTORY: *None*

GOALS:
MD/DO: ☒ INCREASE MOBILITY  ☒ INCREASE ADL  ☒ INCREASE STRENGTH  ☒ DECREASE PAIN

PRECAUTIONS: ☐ CARDIAC  MAX-SBP ____ DBP ____ HR ____
ABOVE BASELINE  ☐ DIABETES: HYPER/HYPOGLYCEMIA  ☐ ORTHOSTASIS
☐ OTHER _____

WEIGHT BEARING:  ☐ WBAT  ☐ TTWB  ☐ NWB
TO: _____

MODALITIES: ☐ ULTRASOUND TO: *LLE x 7 min*
☐ E-STIM  TO: *LLE x 7 min B/L*

☐ FLUID THERAPY  ☐ JOBST  ☐ PARAFFIN
TO: _____
☐ ICE  TO: *10 min to LLE*

☐ HOTPACKS  TO: *10 min to LLE*
☐ EXERCISES  ☐ PROM  ☐ AAROM  ☐ AROM
TO: *B/L LE*
☒ PRE's  ☐ ISOMETRICS  ☐ ISOKINETICS
TO: *B/L LE*
☐ SLIDEBOARD  ☐ PLYOMETRICS  ☐ MODIFIED KNEE BEND
☐ STEPUPS
☐ LUMBAR STABILIZATION  ☐ WILLIAM's  ☐ McKENZIE  ☐ CERVICAL EXERCISES
☐ RELAXATION  ☐ COORDINATION

MANUAL: ☒ CONTRACT RELAX  ☐ CRANIOSACRAL  ☒ JONES/C-STRAIN  ☒ SOFT
TISSUE MOBILIZATION
☒ STRETCHING  ☒ MASSAGE  ☒ MYOF AS RELEASE  ☒ SPRAY/STRETCH
TO: *LE B/L*

EDUCATION: ☒ MOBILITY:  ☐ TRANSFERS  ☒ ADL  ☒ HEP  ☐ ENERGY CONSERV
☐ WORK HARDENING  ☒ BIOMECHANICS  ☐ 1
HANDED TECHNIQUES
☐ GAIT TRAINING  ☐ FINE MOTOR  ☐ COORD/BALANCE
OTHER: _____
_____
_____

ADL-ACTIVITIES OF DAILY LIVING  AAROM-ACTIVE/ASSISTIVERANGEOFMOTION  DBP-
DIASTOLIC BLOOD PRESSURE
SBP-SYSTOLIC BLOOD PRESSURE  HR-HEART RATE  HEP-HOME EXERCISE PROGRAM
NWB-NON-WEIGHT BEARING
PRE's-PROGRESSIVE RESISTIVE EXERCISES  WBAT-WEIGHT BEARING AS TOLERATED
ROM-RANGE OF MOTION

The above is medically necessary to decrease debility and achieve ADL independence. Also to:
☒ decrease pain, ☒ improve strength/endurance, ☒ improve balance coordination, ☒ improve gait,
☒ improve transfers,
Other _____

PHYSICIAN'S SIGNATURE _____ DATE _____

# CASE **31**

# MEDIAL TIBIAL STRESS SYNDROME ("SHIN SPLINTS")

**CC:** Left shin pain

**HPI:** Ms. R is 43 years old and enjoys going for long walks. She complains of left anterior shin pain that hurts when she starts walking, and then feels better if she continues to "push through the pain." After she finishes her walk, however, the shin aches for about 30 minutes. This has been happening for a month. She is healthy and wants to continue walking, but the pain is making this very difficult. No numbness, tingling, or burning. No weakness.

**PMHx:** None

**PSHx:** None

**Meds:** None

**Allergies:** KDA

**Social:** No tobacco. Social EtOH

**ROS:** Noncontributory

## PHYSICAL EXAMINATION

On exam, Ms. R. is a well-developed female who appears younger than her stated age. BP: 110/60, P: 68, RR: 14. She has 5/5 strength, intact sensation, and 2+ patella and Achilles reflexes in the bilateral lower extremities. 2+ distal pulses are palpated bilaterally. There is no swelling or ecchymosis in the lower extremities bilaterally. Tenderness is noted along the medial aspect of the left tibia. Bilateral hyperpronation of the feet is noted.

## Impression
Medial tibial stress syndrome

## Plan
1. X-ray left tibia
2. Orthotics
3. Physical therapy

# PHYSICAL THERAPY

The patient is a 43-year-old female who presents with left medial shin pain that started several weeks ago while walking. The patient went to the physician who found that she has a medial stress fracture to the tibia and was referred to physical therapy.

**Scale:** 6–7/10 pain

**Increase pain:** walking >30 minutes

**Decrease pain:** rest

# RANGE OF MOTION

**Hip**
Hip extension: WNL

**Knee**
Left knee flexion: WNL
Left knee extension: WNL

**Ankle**
Right ankle dorsiflexion: WNL
Left ankle dorsiflexion: −15 degrees

**Joint play**
Talocrural 2/6 left side

**Special tests**
Anterior impingement + to left talocrural

**Manual muscle testing**
WNL

**Neurodynamic assessment**
WNL

**Tight tender points/soft tissue restrictions**
Left: gastroc, anterior tibialis, posterior tibialis, flexor hallucis longus, flexor digitorum longus—trigger points
Left: extensor retinaculum, anterior tibialis, flexor retinaculum—soft tissue restrictions

**Posture**
Pes planus foot left greater than right

**Ergonomics**
WNL

## ASSESSMENT

The patient presents with signs and symptoms consistent with left medial shin pain consistent with medial tibial stress fracture. The patient presents with an increase in symptoms with walking >30 minutes. Trigger points in left gastroc, anterior tibialis, posterior tibialis, flexor hallucis longus, and flexor digitorum longus. Soft tissue restrictions noted in left anterior tibialis, extensor, and flexor retinaculum.

### Plan

Self–myofascial release/corrective flexibility/corrective exercises/corrective manual therapy/modalities

### Self–Myofascial Release

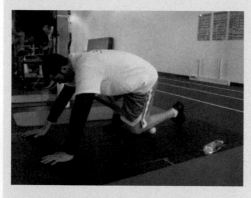

**FIGURE 31.1A.** Tennis ball: left anterior tibialis

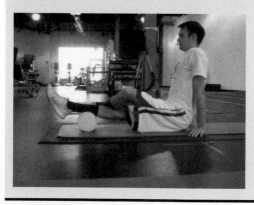

**FIGURE 31.1B.** Foam roll: left gastroc

# Corrective Flexibility

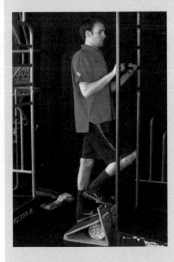

**FIGURE 31.2A.** Static: left gastroc

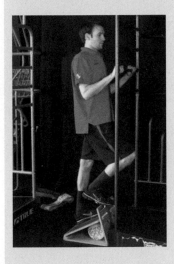

**FIGURE 31.2B.** Active: bilateral gastroc

(*continued*)

## Corrective Flexibility (*continued*)

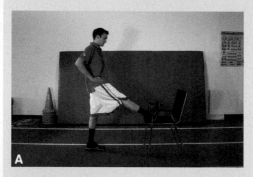

**FIGURE    31.3(A–C).**    Active: bilateral hamstrings 3D on chair

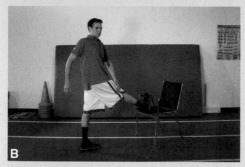

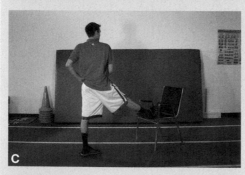

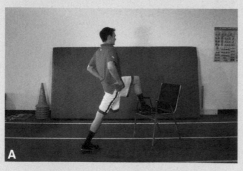

**FIGURE 31.4(A–C).** Active: bilateral hip flexor 3D on chair

(*continued*)

## Corrective Flexibility (*continued*)

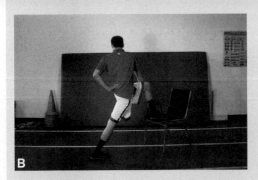

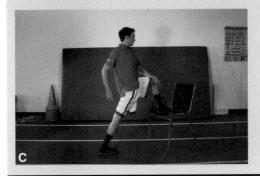

## Corrective Exercise

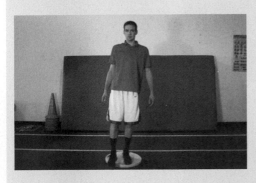

**FIGURE 31.5A.** BAPS: clockwise/counter clockwise

*(continued)*

# Corrective Exercise (*continued*)

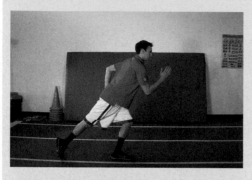

**FIGURE 31.5B.** Running techniques on single leg

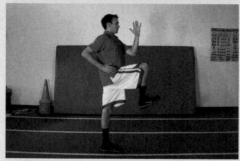

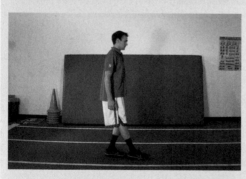

**FIGURE 31.5C.** Balance reach: 3D

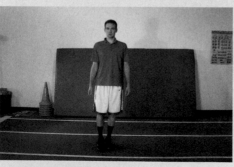

(*continued*)

## Corrective Exercise (*continued*)

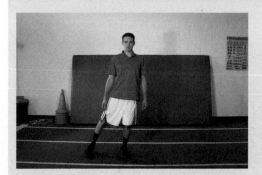

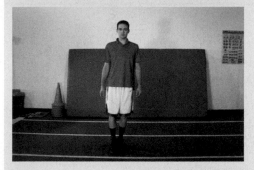

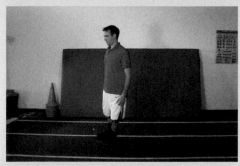

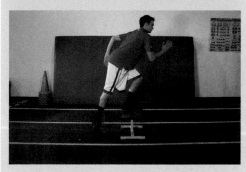

**FIGURE 31.5D.** Step-up technique

(*continued*)

## Corrective Exercise (*continued*)

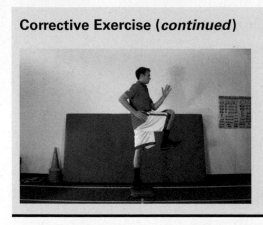

## Manual Therapy

1. Warming technique: left gastroc, anterior tibialis,
2. Inhibitory technique: left flexor digitorum longus, flexor hallucis longus, and posterior tibialis
3. Activation technique: left anterior tibialis proximal attachment and medial gastroc
4. Elongation technique: left flexor and extensor retinaculum, anterior tibialis

## Modalities

1. Ice medial shin prn

## Home Exercise Program

1. Tennis ball: left anterior tibialis
2. Foam roll: left gastroc
3. Static: anterior tibialis left
4. Static: gastroc left
5. Active: hamstring left

Orthopedic and Rehabilitation Associates
Orthopedic Street
Omaha, OH
(555) 555-5555
Fax. (666) 666-7777

PATIENT: _Ms. R_
DATE: _2009_

## ORTHOPAEDIC REHABILITATION PRESCRIPTION

REHAB THERAPIES    ☒ PT    ☐ OT    ☐ SESSIONS/WK _2_
TOTAL _12_

☒ NEW DIAGNOSIS    ☐ RE-EVALUATION    ☒ OUTPATIENT

DIAGNOSIS1 _Medial Tibial Stress Syndrome_
   ICD _____

DIAGNOSIS2 _____
   ICD _____

PREGNANT? ☐ YES ☒ NO      PERTINENTMEDICALHISTORY: _None_

GOALS:
MD/DO: ☒ INCREASE MOBILITY ☒ INCREASE ADL ☒ INCREASE STRENGTH ☒ DECREASE PAIN

PRECAUTIONS: ☐ CARDIAC    MAX-SBP ____ DBP ____ HR ____
ABOVE BASELINE    ☐ DIABETES: HYPER/HYPOGLYCEMIA ☐ ORTHOSTASIS
☐ OTHER _____
WEIGHT BEARING:    ☐ WBAT    ☐ TTWB    ☐ NWB
   TO: _____
MODALITIES: ☐ ULTRASOUND TO: _LLE x 7 min_____
     ☐ E-STIM    TO: _LLE x 7 min B/L_____

     ☐ FLUID THERAPY    ☐ JOBST    ☐ PARAFFIN
   TO: _____
     ☐ ICE    TO: _10 min to LLE_

     ☐ HOTPACKS    TO: _10 min to LLE_
     ☐ EXERCISES ☐ PROM ☐ AAROM ☐ AROM
   TO: _B/L LE_
     ☒ PRE's ☐ ISOMETRICS ☐ ISOKINETICS
   TO. _B/L LE_
     ☐ SLIDEBOARD ☐ PLYOMETRICS ☐ MODIFIED KNEE BEND
☐ STEPUPS
☐ LUMBAR STABILIZATION ☐ WILLIAM's ☐ McKENZIE ☐ CERVICAL EXERCISES
☐ RELAXATION ☐ COORDINATION
MANUAL: ☒ CONTRACT RELAX ☐ CRANIOSACRAL ☒ JONES/C-STRAIN ☒ SOFT
TISSUE MOBILIZATION
     ☒ STRETCHING ☒ MASSAGE ☒ MYOF AS RELEASE ☒ SPRAY/STRETCH
   TO: _LE B/L_
EDUCATION: ☒ MOBILITY: ☐ TRANSFERS ☒ ADL ☒ HEP ☐ ENERGY CONSERV
☐ WORK HARDENING ☒ BIOMECHANICS ☐ 1
HANDED TECHNIQUES
☐ GAIT TRAINING ☐ FINE MOTOR ☐ COORD/BALANCE
OTHER: _____
_____
_____

ADL-ACTIVITIES OF DAILY LIVING    AAROM-ACTIVE/ASSISTIVERANGEOFMOTION   DBP-
DIASTOLIC BLOOD PRESSURE
SBP-SYSTOLIC BLOOD PRESSURE    HR-HEART RATE    HEP-HOME EXERCISE PROGRAM
NWB-NON-WEIGHT BEARING
PRE's-PROGRESSIVE RESISTIVE EXERCISES    WBAT-WEIGHT BEARING AS TOLERATED
ROM-RANGE OF MOTION

The above is medically necessary to decrease debility and achieve ADL independence. Also to:
☒ decrease pain, ☒ improve strength/endurance, ☒ improve balance coordination, ☒ improve gait,
☒ improve transfers,
Other _____

PHYSICIAN'S SIGNATURE _____ DATE _____

# PART **10**

## ANKLE AND FOOT

# CASE 32

# ACHILLES TENDONITIS

**CC:** Achilles pain

**HPI:** Ms. B is 34 years old and plays soccer on the weekends. Over the last 3 weeks she has noted increasing pain in her left Achilles tendon when she tries to run. Sometimes the pain is also present when she walks. The pain is close to the heel. No numbness, tingling, or burning. No weakness. She has not noted this sort of pain before. The pain is 8/10 when she runs and 0/10 when she is sitting.

**PMHx:** None

**PSHx:** None

**Meds:** None

**Allergies:** NKDA

**Social:** No tobacco; social EtOH

**ROS:** Noncontributory

## PHYSICAL EXAMINATION

On exam, Ms. B is a well-developed female who appears her stated age. BP: 100/62, P: 68, RR: 14. She has 5/5 strength, intact sensation, and 2+ patella and Achilles reflexes in the bilateral lower extremities. 2+ distal pulses are palpated bilaterally. She has her typical pain when performing single leg toe raises on the left. Tenderness is noted over the distal portion of the Achilles tendon as it inserts into the calcaneus. Negative Thompson test bilaterally. Ms. B does not exhibit hyperpronation on either foot.

**253**

## Impression

Achilles tendonitis

**Plan**

**1.** Physical therapy

# PHYSICAL THERAPY

The patient is a 34-year-old female who presents with left Achilles pain that started 3 weeks ago while running. The patient is a soccer player and the pain progressively got worse. The patient went to her medical doctor who referred her to physical therapy,

**Scale:** 8/10 pain

**Increase pain:** running and prolonged walking

**Decrease pain:** sitting

## Range of Motion

**Hip**

Hip extension: WNL

**Knee**

Left knee flexion: WNL

Left knee extension: WNL

**Ankle**

Right ankle dorsiflexion: WNL

Left ankle dorsiflexion: –10 degrees with pain

**Joint play**

WNL

**Special tests**

SLR – (but restricted hamstrings noted)

**Manual muscle testing**

WNL

**Neurodynamic assessment**

WNL

**Tight tender points/soft tissue restrictions**

Left: gastroc, posterior tibialis, flexor hallucis longus, flexor digitorum longus—trigger points

Left: gastroc, flexor digitorum longus, plantar fascia, hamstrings, flexor retinaculum—soft tissue restrictions

**Posture**

WNL

**Ergonomics**

WNL

# ASSESSMENT

The patient presents with signs and symptoms consistent with Achilles tendonitis. She presents with an increase in symptoms with running and prolonged walking. Trigger points in left gastroc, posterior tibialis, flexor hallucis longus, and flexor digitorum longus. Soft tissue restrictions noted in gastroc, flexor digitorum longus, plantar fascia, hamstrings, and flexor retinaculum.

## Plan

Self–myofascial release/corrective flexibility/corrective exercises/corrective manual therapy/modalities

### Self–Myofascial Release

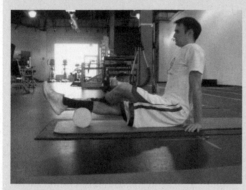

**FIGURE 32.1.** Tennis ball: left gastroc.

### Corrective Flexibility

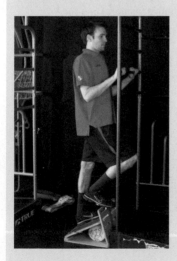

**FIGURE 32.2A.** Static: left gastroc.

(*continued*)

## Corrective Flexibility (*continued*)

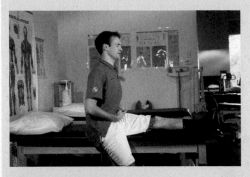

**FIGURE 32.2B.** Static: left hamstring on the table.

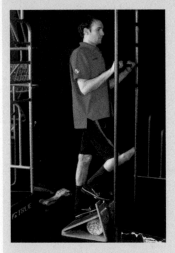

**FIGURE 32.2C.** Active: bilateral gastroc.

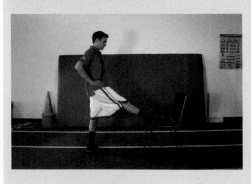

**FIGURE 32.2D.** Active: bilateral hamstrings 3D on chair.

(*continued*)

## Corrective Flexibility (*continued*)

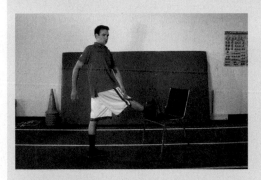

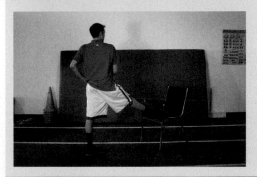

## Corrective Exercise

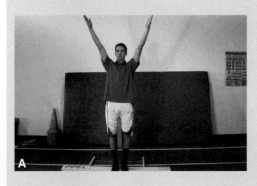

**FIGURE 32.3(A–B).** Progressive hamstring.

(*continued*)

## Corrective Exercise (*continued*)

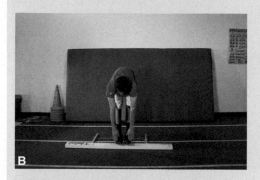

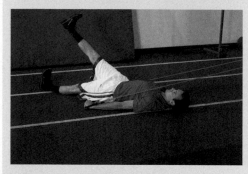

**FIGURE 32.4.** Straight leg raise with core activation.

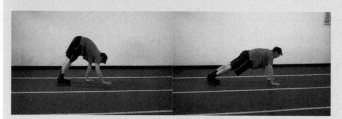

**FIGURE 32.5.** Walkouts

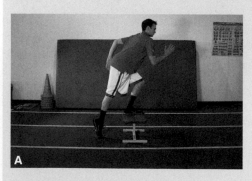

**FIGURE 32.6(A–B).** Step-up technique.

(*continued*)

## Corrective Exercise (*continued*)

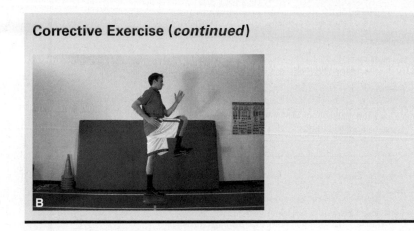

## Manual Therapy

1. Warming technique: left gastroc, hamstring
2. Inhibitory technique: left flexor digitorum longus, flexor hallucis longus, and posterior tibialis
3. Elongation technique: left flexor retinaculum, flexor digitorum longus, flexor hallucis longus, plantar fascia, hamstring, and posterior tibialis

## Modalities

1. Ice to the Achilles attachment prn

## Home Exercise Program

1. Tennis ball: left gastroc
2. Static: hamstring left on table

Orthopedic and Rehabilitation Associates
Orthopedic Street
Omaha, OH
(555) 555-5555
Fax. (666) 666-7777

PATIENT: *Ms. B*
DATE: *2009*

## ORTHOPAEDIC REHABILITATION PRESCRIPTION

| REHAB THERAPIES | ☒ PT | ☐ OT | ☐ SESSIONS/WK *2* |
| --- | --- | --- | --- |

TOTAL *12*

☒ NEW DIAGNOSIS    ☐ RE-EVALUATION    ☒ OUTPATIENT

DIAGNOSIS1 *Achilles Tendonitis*
   ICD _____

DIAGNOSIS2 _____
   ICD _____

PREGNANT? ☐ YES  ☒ NO        PERTINENTMEDICALHISTORY: *DM*

GOALS:
MD/DO: ☒ INCREASE MOBILITY  ☒ INCREASE ADL  ☒ INCREASE STRENGTH  ☒ DECREASE PAIN

PRECAUTIONS: ☐ CARDIAC    MAX-SBP____ DBP____ HR____
ABOVE BASELINE    ☐ DIABETES: HYPER/HYPOGLYCEMIA  ☐ ORTHOSTASIS
☐ OTHER _____

WEIGHT BEARING:  ☐ WBAT   ☐ TTWB   ☐ NWB
   TO: _____

MODALITIES: ☐ ULTRASOUND TO: *RLE x 7 min*
      ☐ E-STIM   TO: *RLE x 7 min B/L*

   ☐ FLUID THERAPY    ☐ JOBST    ☐ PARAFFIN
TO: _____
   ☐ ICE   TO: *10 min to LLE*

   ☐ HOTPACKS   TO: *10 min to LLE*
   ☐ EXERCISES  ☐ PROM  ☐ AAROM  ☐ AROM
TO: *B/L LE*
   ☒ PRE's  ☐ ISOMETRICS  ☐ ISOKINETICS
TO: *B/L LE*
   ☐ SLIDEBOARD  ☐ PLYOMETRICS  ☐ MODIFIED KNEE BEND
☐ STEPUPS
☐ LUMBAR STABILIZATION  ☐ WILLIAM's  ☐ McKENZIE  ☐ CERVICAL EXERCISES
☐ RELAXATION  ☐ COORDINATION

MANUAL: ☒ CONTRACT RELAX  ☐ CRANIOSACRAL  ☒ JONES/C-STRAIN  ☒ SOFT
TISSUE MOBILIZATION
      ☒ STRETCHING  ☒ MASSAGE  ☒ MYOF AS RELEASE  ☒ SPRAY/STRETCH
   TO: *LE B/L*

EDUCATION: ☒ MOBILITY:  ☐ TRANSFERS  ☒ ADL  ☒ HEP  ☐ ENERGY CONSERV
   ☐ WORK HARDENING  ☒ BIOMECHANICS  ☐ 1
HANDED TECHNIQUES
   ☐ GAIT TRAINING  ☐ FINE MOTOR  ☐ COORD/BALANCE
OTHER: _____
_____
_____

ADL-ACTIVITIES OF DAILY LIVING    AAROM-ACTIVE/ASSISTIVERANGEOFMOTION   DBP-
DIASTOLIC BLOOD PRESSURE
SBP-SYSTOLIC BLOOD PRESSURE    HR-HEART RATE    HEP-HOME EXERCISE PROGRAM
NWB-NON-WEIGHT BEARING
PRE's-PROGRESSIVE RESISTIVE EXERCISES    WBAT-WEIGHT BEARING AS TOLERATED
ROM-RANGE OF MOTION

The above is medically necessary to decrease debility and achieve ADL independence. Also to:
☒ decrease pain, ☒ improve strength/endurance, ☒ improve balance coordination, ☒ improve gait,
☒ improve transfers,
Other _____

PHYSICIAN'S SIGNATURE _____ DATE _____

# CASE **33**

## ANKLE SPRAIN

**CC:** "I sprained my ankle."

**HPI:** Mr. U is 44 years old and was stepping off the curb 2 days ago and "fell over" his right ankle. The lateral aspect of the ankle has been painful ever since. He is able to place weight on the ankle and has been ambulating with a limp since the accident. He denies any locking or catching of the ankle. The pain is 4/10 intensity and is more painful with weight-bearing. He did not go to the ER, but is coming to the office because the pain has not gotten better. No numbness, tingling, or burning.

**PMHx:** DM type II

**PSHx:** None

**Meds:** Glucophage

**Allergies:** NKDA

**Social:** No tobacco. Social EtOH

**ROS:** Noncontributory

## PHYSICAL EXAMINATION

On exam, Mr. U is an overweight male who appears his stated age. BP: 142/88, P: 77, RR: 14. He has 5/5 strength, intact sensation, and 2+ patella and Achilles reflexes in the bilateral lower extremities. 2+ distal pulses are palpated bilaterally. He has an antalgic gait, favoring his left side. Tenderness is noted along his right ATFL. Anterior drawer test and talar tilt tests are negative bilaterally. Minimal swelling is noted in the right ankle. No bony tenderness is found. No hyperpronation is noted bilaterally.

## Impression

Grade I ankle sprain

## Plan

1. PRICE
2. Physical therapy

## PHYSICAL THERAPY

The patient is a 44-year-old male who sprained his right ankle while stepping off a curb last week. The patient went to the physician who did a physical exam and referred the patient to physical therapy.

**Scale:** 4/10 pain

**Increase pain:** weight bearing; ankle inversion and plantar flexion

**Decrease pain:** sitting

## Range of Motion

**Hip**

Hip extension: WNL

**Knee**

Left knee flexion: WNL

Left knee extension: WNL

**Ankle**

Left ankle dorsiflexion: WNL

Right ankle dorsiflexion: −10 degrees with pain

Right ankle inversion: 15 degrees with pain

Right ankle plantar flexion: WNL with pain

**Joint play**

Empty

**Special tests**

Anterior draw +

**Manual muscle testing**

WNL

**Neurodynamic assessment**

WNL

**Tight tender points/soft tissue restrictions**

Right gastroc, peroneus longus/brevis—trigger points

Right: gastroc, flexor digitorum longus, plantar fascia, psoas, gluteus medius, extensor retinaculum—soft tissue restrictions

**Posture**

WNL

**Ergonomics**

WNL

## ASSESSMENT

The patient presents with signs and symptoms consistent with right ankle sprain. The patient presents with an increase in symptoms with weight bearing, plantar flexion, and inversion. Trigger points in right gastroc, peroneus longus/brevis. Soft tissue restrictions noted in gastroc, flexor digitorum longus, plantar fascia, psoas, gluteus medius, and flexor retinaculum.

### Plan

Self–myofascial release/corrective flexibility/corrective exercises/corrective manual therapy/modalities

## Self–Myofascial Release

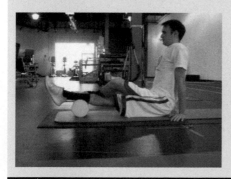

**FIGURE 33.1** Tennis ball: right gastroc.

## Corrective Flexibility

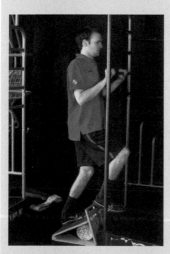

**FIGURE 33.2** Active: soleus.

(*continued*)

## Corrective Flexibility (*continued*)

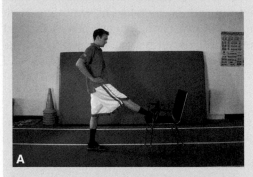

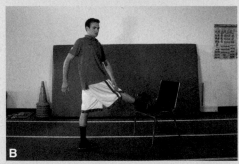

**FIGURE 33.3(A–C).** Active: hamstring 3D.

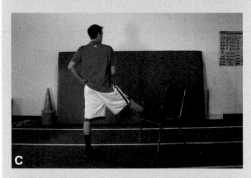

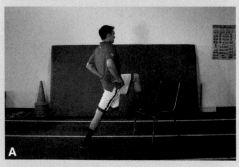

**FIGURE 33.4(A–C).** Active: hip flexor 3D.

(*continued*)

## Corrective Flexibility (*continued*)

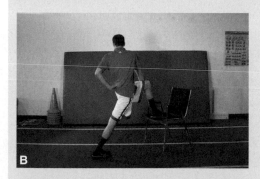

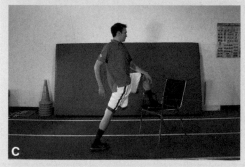

## Corrective Exercise

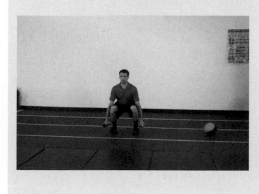

**FIGURE 33.5A.** Squat: parallel stance.

*(continued)*

## Corrective Exercise (*continued*)

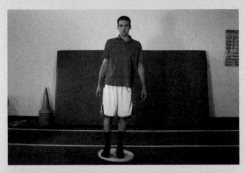

**FIGURE 33.5B**. BAPS clockwise/counter clockwise.

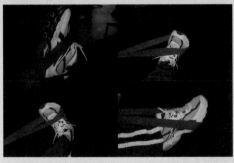

**FIGURE 33.5C**. Resisted dorsi-flexion/eversion/inversion/plantar flexion—fast and short ROM.

## Manual Therapy

1. Warming technique: right gastroc
2. Activation technique: right peroneus longus; anterior tibialis
3. Inhibitory technique: right psoas; gluteus medius
4. Elongation technique: right gastroc; psoas

## Modalities

1. Ice to the ankle prn

## Home Exercise Program

1. Tennis ball: right gastroc
2. Active: right soleus

Orthopedic and Rehabilitation Associates
Orthopedic Street
Omaha, OH
(555) 555-5555
Fax. (666) 666-7777

PATIENT: *Mr. U*
DATE: *2009*

## ORTHOPAEDIC REHABILITATION PRESCRIPTION

*REHAB THERAPIES*      ☒ PT        ☐ OT        ☐ SESSIONS/WK _*2*_
TOTAL *12*

☒ NEW DIAGNOSIS        ☐ RE-EVALUATION        ☒ OUTPATIENT

DIAGNOSIS1 *Ankle sprain*
    ICD _____

DIAGNOSIS2 _____
    ICD _____

PREGNANT? ☐ YES  ☒ NO          PERTINENTMEDICALHISTORY: *None*

GOALS:
MD/DO: ☒ INCREASE MOBILITY ☒ INCREASE ADL ☒ INCREASE STRENGTH ☒ DECREASE PAIN

PRECAUTIONS: ☐ CARDIAC      MAX-SBP____ DBP___ HR ____
ABOVE BASELINE      ☐ DIABETES: HYPER/HYPOGLYCEMIA ☐ ORTHOSTASIS
☐ OTHER _____
WEIGHT BEARING:      ☐ WBAT      ☐ TTWB      ☐ NWB
    TO: _____
MODALITIES: ☐ ULTRASOUND TO: *LLE x 7 min*
            ☐ E-STIM      TO: *LLE x 7 min B/L*

        ☐ FLUID THERAPY      ☐ JOBST      ☐ PARAFFIN
    TO: _____
        ☐ ICE      TO: *10 min to LLE*

        ☐ HOTPACKS      TO: *10 min to LLE*
        ☐ EXERCISES ☐ PROM ☐ AAROM ☐ AROM
    TO: *B/L LE*
        ☒ PRE's    ☐ ISOMETRICS    ☐ ISOKINETICS
    TO: *B/L LE*
        ☐ SLIDEBOARD ☐ PLYOMETRICS ☐ MODIFIED KNEE BEND
☐ STEPUPS
☐ LUMBAR STABILIZATION ☐ WILLIAM's ☐ McKENZIE ☐ CERVICAL EXERCISES
☐ RELAXATION ☐ COORDINATION
MANUAL: ☒ CONTRACT RELAX ☐ CRANIOSACRAL ☒ JONES/C-STRAIN ☒ SOFT
TISSUE MOBILIZATION
        ☒ STRETCHING ☐ MASSAGE ☒ MYOF AS RELEASE ☒ SPRAY/STRETCH
    TO: *LE B/L*
EDUCATION: ☒ MOBILITY: ☐ TRANSFERS ☒ ADL ☒ HEP ☐ ENERGY CONSERV
    ☐ WORK HARDENING ☒ BIOMECHANICS ☐ 1
HANDED TECHNIQUES
    ☒ GAIT TRAINING ☐ FINE MOTOR ☐ COORD/BALANCE
OTHER: _____

ADL-ACTIVITIES OF DAILY LIVING      AAROM-ACTIVE/ASSISTIVERANGEOFMOTION   DBP-
DIASTOLIC BLOOD PRESSURE
SBP-SYSTOLIC BLOOD PRESSURE   HR-HEART RATE   HEP-HOME EXERCISE PROGRAM
NWB-NON-WEIGHT BEARING
PRE's-PROGRESSIVE RESISTIVE EXERCISES   WBAT-WEIGHT BEARING AS TOLERATED
ROM-RANGE OF MOTION

The above is medically necessary to decrease debility and achieve ADL independence. Also to:
☒ decrease pain, ☒ improve strength/endurance, ☒ improve balance coordination, ☒ improve gait,
☒ improve transfers,
Other _____

PHYSICIAN'S SIGNATURE _____ DATE _____

# PLANTAR FASCIITIS

**CC:** Heel pain

**HPI:** Mr. N is 38 years old and complains of 3-week history of left heel pain. The pain is worst when he first gets up in the morning and takes his first step. The pain is also exacerbated when he stands up after sitting for a while. As he walks, the pain dissipates at first, but if he keeps walking then the pain returns. No lower leg pain. No numbness, tingling, or weakness. No trauma. The pain began gradually.

**PMHx:** None

**PSHx:** None

**Meds:** Glucophage

**Allergies:** NKDA

**Social:** No tobacco. Social EtOH

**ROS:** Noncontributory

## PHYSICAL EXAMINATION

On exam, Mr. N is in no acute distress and appears his stated age. BP: 138/78, P: 70, RR: 14. He has 5/5 strength, intact sensation, and 2+ patella and Achilles reflexes in the bilateral lower extremities. 2+ distal pulses are palpated bilaterally. He exhibits bilateral hyperpronation. Tenderness is noted on the medial aspect of his left calcaneus. Passive dorsiflexion of the left foot is uncomfortable for him. No swelling is noted. The pain is 5/10 in the morning when he takes his first few steps. He is not taking any pain medications.

## Impression

Plantar fasciitis

## Plan

1. X-ray bilateral feet
2. Orthotics
3. Physical therapy

# PHYSICAL THERAPY

The patient is a 38-year-old male who presents with left heel pain that started 3 weeks ago. The onset of pain was insidious. He went to the physician who referred him to physical therapy.

**Scale:** 5/10 pain

**Increase pain:** mornings; walking barefoot; prolonged sitting to standing

**Decrease pain:** sitting

## Range of Motion

**Hip**

Hip extension: WNL

**Knee**

Left knee flexion: WNL

Left knee extension: WNL

**Ankle**

Right ankle dorsiflexion: WNL

Left ankle dorsiflexion: –5 degrees with pain

**Manual muscle testing**

WNL

**Neurodynamic assessment**

WNL

**Tight tender points/soft tissue restrictions**

Left: gastroc; posterior tibialis; flexor hallucis longus/brevis; flexor digitorum longus/brevis; quadratus plantae; plantar fascia—trigger points

Left: gastroc, flexor digitorum longus/brevis, plantar fascia; flexor hallucis longus/brevis—soft tissue restrictions

**Posture**

WNL

**Ergonomics**

WNL

# ASSESSMENT

The patient presents with signs and symptoms consistent with left plantar fasciitis. The patient presents with an increase in symptoms walking barefoot, first thing in the morning, and prolonged sitting to stand. Trigger points in left gastroc, posterior tibialis, flexor hallucis longus/brevis, flexor digitorum longus/brevis, quadratus plantae, and plantar fascia. Soft tissue restrictions noted in left gastroc, flexor digitorum longus/brevis, plantar fascia, and flexor hallucis longus/brevis.

## Plan

Self–myofascial release/corrective flexibility/corrective exercises/corrective manual therapy/modalities

### Self–Myofascial Release

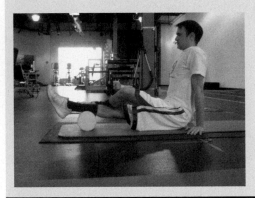

**FIGURE 34.1.** Foam roll: left gastroc. Golf ball: left plantar fascia.

### Corrective Flexibility

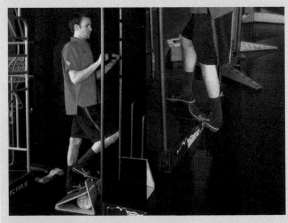

**FIGURE 34.2A.** Static: two way: gastroc/soleus with toe dorsiflexion against wall (knee straight to knee bent).

(*continued*)

## Corrective Flexibility (*continued*)

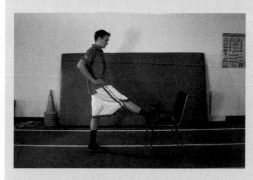

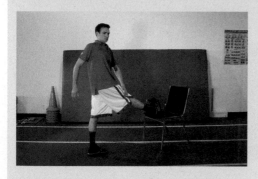

**FIGURE 34.2B.** Active: hamstring 3D.

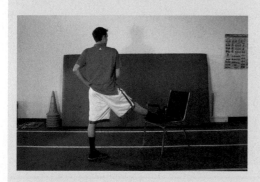

(*continued*)

## Corrective Flexibility

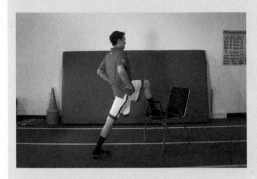

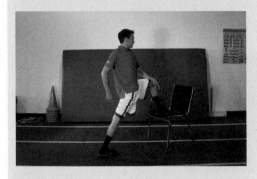

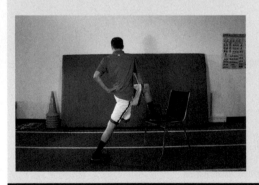

**FIGURE 34.2C.** Active: hip flexor 3D.

## Corrective Exercise

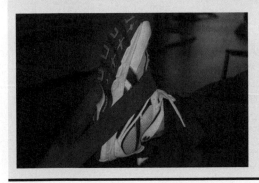

**FIGURE 34.3.** Resisted dorsiflexion: theraband (fast and short range).

## Manual Therapy

1. Warming technique: left gastroc
2. Activation technique: left anterior tibialis
3. Inhibitory technique: left psoas; gastroc/soleus/flexor digitorum/hallucis
4. Elongation technique: right gastroc; psoas; flexor digitorum longus/brevis and flexor hallucis longus/brevis

## Modalities

1. Ice prn
2. Ultrasound to plantar fascia prn

## Home Exercise Program

1. Foam roll: left gastroc
2. Golf ball: left plantar fascia

Orthopedic and Rehabilitation Associates
Orthopedic Street
Omaha, OH
(555) 555-5555
Fax. (666) 666-7777

PATIENT: _Mr. N_
DATE: _2009_

## ORTHOPAEDIC REHABILITATION PRESCRIPTION

**REHAB THERAPIES**    ☒ PT    ☐ OT    ☐ SESSIONS/WK _2_
TOTAL _12_

☐ NEW DIAGNOSIS    ☒ RE-EVALUATION    ☒ OUTPATIENT

DIAGNOSIS1 _Plantar Fasciitis_
    ICD _____

DIAGNOSIS2 _____
    ICD _____

PREGNANT? ☐ YES ☒ NO     PERTINENT MEDICAL HISTORY: _None_

GOALS:
MD/DO: ☒ INCREASE MOBILITY ☒ INCREASE ADL ☒ INCREASE STRENGTH ☒ DECREASE PAIN

PRECAUTIONS: ☐ CARDIAC    MAX-SBP _____ DBP _____ HR _____
ABOVE BASELINE    ☐ DIABETES: HYPER/HYPOGLYCEMIA ☐ ORTHOSTASIS
☐ OTHER _____
WEIGHT BEARING:    ☐ WBAT    ☐ TTWB    ☐ NWB
    TO: _____
MODALITIES: ☐ ULTRASOUND TO: _Left foot x 7 min_
         ☐ E-STIM     TO: _Left foot x 7 min B/L_
B/L _____
    ☐ FLUID THERAPY    ☐ JOBST    ☐ PARAFFIN
    TO: _____
    ☐ ICE    TO: _10 min to left foot_
B/L _____
    ☐ HOTPACKS    TO: _10 min to left foot_
    ☐ EXERCISES ☐ PROM ☐ AAROM ☐ AROM
    TO: _B/L LE_
    ☒ PRE's ☐ ISOMETRICS ☐ ISOKINETICS
    TO: _B/L LE_
    ☐ SLIDEBOARD ☐ PLYOMETRICS ☐ MODIFIED KNEE BEND
☐ STEPUPS
☐ LUMBAR STABILIZATION ☐ WILLIAM's ☐ McKENZIE ☐ CERVICAL EXERCISES
☐ RELAXATION ☐ COORDINATION
MANUAL: ☒ CONTRACT RELAX ☐ CRANIOSACRAL ☒ JONES/C-STRAIN ☒ SOFT
TISSUE MOBILIZATION
    ☒ STRETCHING ☒ MASSAGE ☒ MYOFAS RELEASE ☒ SPRAY/STRETCH
    TO: _LE B/L_
EDUCATION: ☒ MOBILITY: ☐ TRANSFERS ☒ ADL ☒ HEP ☐ ENERGY CONSERV

☐ WORK HARDENING ☒ BIOMECHANICS ☐ 1 HANDED TECHNIQUES

☐ GAIT TRAINING ☐ FINE MOTOR ☐ COORD/BALANCE

OTHER: _____

The above is medically necessary to decrease debility and achieve ADL independence. Also to:
☒ decrease pain, ☒ improve strength/endurance, ☒ improve balance coordination, ☒ improve gait,
☒ improve transfers,
Other _____

PHYSICIAN'S SIGNATURE _____ DATE _____

# INDEX

Page number in *italics* denotes figures.